The Authorities

~ *Powerful Wisdom from Leaders in the Field* ~

WILMA DAVID AGUILA

Award Winning Author

AuthoritiesPress

Publisher
Authorities Press
Markham, ON
Canada

Printed in the United States and Canada.

FOREWORD

Experts are to be admired for their knowledge, but they often remain unrecognized by the general public because they save their information and insights for paying customers and clients. There are many experts in a given field, but their impact is limited to the handful of people with whom they work.

Unlike experts, authorities share their knowledge and expertise far more broadly, so they make a big impact on the world. Authorities become known and admired as leading experts and, as such, typically do very well economically and professionally. Most authorities are also mature enough to know that part of the joy of monetary success is the accompanying moral and spiritual obligation to give back.

Many people want to learn and work with well-respected and generous authorities, but don't always know where to find them. They may be known to their peers, or within a specific community, but have not had the opportunity to reach a wider audience. At one time, they might have submitted a proposal to the For Dummies or Chicken Soup for the Soul series of books, but it's now almost impossible to get accepted as a new author in such branded book series.

It is more than fitting that Raymond Aaron, an internationally known and respected authority in his own right, would be the one to recognize the need for a new venue in which authorities could share their considerable knowledge with readers everywhere. As the only author ever to be included in both of the book series mentioned above, Raymond has had the opportunity to give back and he understands how crucial it is for authorities to have a platform from which to share their expertise.

I have known and worked with Raymond for a number of years and consider him a valued friend and talented coach. He knows how to spot talented and knowledgeable people and he desires to see them prosper. Over the years, success coaching and speaking engagements around the world have made it possible for Raymond to meet many of these talented authorities. He recognizes and relates to their passion and enthusiasm for what they do, as well as their desire to share what they know. He tells me that's why he created this new nonfiction branded book series, The Authorities.

Dr. Nido Qubein
President, High Point University

TABLE OF CONTENTS

Introduction V

The Love Drug 1
Wilma David Aguila

Step Into Greatness 23
Les Brown

Branding Small Business 33
Raymond Aaron

Sex, Love and Relationships 45
Dr. John Gray

Your Life Energy 51
Amal Indi

Nobody Got Time For That! 65
Ursula Garrett

Simple Steps for Big Results in Boosting Heart Health 83
Ralston Powell

Break Free From Your Pain Cycle 95
Seema Giri

Find Your True Self with Yoga and Pole 123
Lynne Niepage

The Modern Healer 135
Herman Siu and Martin Siu

Coping with Cancer 153
Yvonne Abou-Nader

Purpose and Living Your Passion Cure 171
Ron Bell

INTRODUCTION

This book introduces you to *The Authorities* — individuals who have distinguished themselves in life and in business. Authorities make a big impact on the world. Authorities are leaders in their chosen fields. Authorities typically do very well financially, and are evolved enough to know that part of the joy of monetary success is the accompanying social, moral and spiritual obligation to give back.

Authorities are not just outstanding. They are also known to be outstanding.

This additional element begins to explain the difference between two strategic business and life concepts — one that seems great, but isn't, and the other that fills in the essential missing gap of the first.

The first concept is "the expert."

What is an expert? The real definition is …

EXPERT: *a person who knows stuff*

People who have attained a very senior academic degree (like a PhD or an MD) definitely know stuff. People who read voraciously and retain what they read definitely know stuff. Unfortunately, just because you know stuff does not mean that anyone respects the fact that you do. Even though some experts are successful, alas, most are not — because knowing stuff is not enough.

Well, then, what is the missing piece?

What the expert lacks, "the authority" has. The authority both knows stuff and is known to know stuff. So, more simply …

AUTHORITY: *a person who is known as an expert*

The difference is not subtle. The difference is not merely semantic. The difference is enormous.

When it comes to this subject, there are actually three categories in which people fall:

- People who don't know much and are unsuccessful in life and in business. Most people fall in this category.

- People who know stuff, but still don't leave much of a footprint in the world. There are a lot of people like this.

- Experts who are also *known* as experts become authorities and authorities are always wondrously successful. Authorities are able to contribute more to humanity through both their chosen work and their giving back.

This book is about the highest category, The Authorities — people who have reached the peak in their field and are known as such.

You will definitely know some of *The Authorities* in this book, especially since there are some world-famous ones. Others are just as exceptional, but you may not yet know about them. Our featured author, Wilma David Aguila, is one of these authors. Wilma is a free sprit who takes life in stride. She did not come from humble beginnings. In fact, it was quite the contrary. Hers was a privileged childhood surrounded by the finer things in life, but she elected instead to abandon those luxuries and leave home. Her objective? Learn more about herself, about people and cultures. She did so with such passion that she left all behind in search of real life experiences she could use to fulfill her desire to help others. Wilma is a World Traveller interested in culture, lifestyle and understanding the human sprit and inner strength. She is passionate about helping others and has donated a lot of time and resources to charitable causes. Wilma has a Chemical Engineering degree and is also an

Entrepreneur. As a business owner she has helped many people change their outlook and perspective on life. She settled in Toronto and is the mother of an independent son.

Over the course of her life, Wilma has been fortunate enough to have had many experiences which taught her a lot of skills and lessons that made her the strong woman she is today. She's followed the motto that "will conquers all." If there is will then there is always a way, a resolution to all life's challenges. She has seen and observed that intensely personal stressors and many physical and emotional obstacles dominate our minds on a frequent basis. During her growing up years, her daily routine was to read a motivational quote each day. This became a habit to her--not just to read the quotes but practice them and share them with others. So, she became passionate about helping, giving, listening and motivating people.

It is Wilma's belief that we are all responsible to make choices in our lives. And she made the choice to redirect her life energy towards helping and motivating people on a metaphysical level.

They are *The Authorities*. Learn from them. Connect with them. Let them uplift you. Learning from them and working with them is the secret ingredient for success which may well allow you to rise to the level of Authority soon.

To be considered for inclusion in a subsequent edition of The Authorities, register to attend a future event at www.aaron.com/events where you will be interviewed and considered.

The Love Drug

Your Lifetime Supply of Metaphysical Pharmaceuticals

WILMA DAVID AGUILA

F irst of all, let me begin by saying I am an advocate of mental wellness and healthy living. In my sixteen years in Canada, I have been privileged to have worked in the pharmaceutical industry, innovating and developing drugs, and in pharmacies where I've had direct interaction with patients. I've learned through these interactions how wide a knowledge gap exists in regard to the awareness of the medicines we take. There's a gap with respect to what a medicine's focus and intention is relative to what the patient may want it to be. Interesting assumptions are made about what the medication may offer, sometimes beyond what the manufacturer intended, all in the search for normalcy and wellbeing.

I'm sure you know of someone who at some time or another resorted to the use of synthetic drugs to self-medicate. For example, some may use pain medications to deal with feelings of heartache or pain associated with failure, fear, anxiety or let-down. Sleeping pills may be used beyond treatment for insomnia, to deal with anxiety or stress. I've encountered people who believe an elevated heart rate that recurs has to be a symptom of a disease, when a little prodding reveals stress as the main culprit. Let's not forget the power of the internet, and how many of us use it to self-diagnose: perhaps the most detrimental factor that drives self-medicating.

The truth is that most people fail to listen to and put faith into the power of their inner voice and its influence on wellness and self-care. In this context, self-care refers to any necessary human regulatory function under an individual's control. There is no intention here to contradict the use of pharmaceutical drugs to treat a true condition or ailment as diagnosed by a medical practitioner, rather it's my intent to emphasise an awareness of metaphysics, and adopting it as a way of life. This chapter will explore a system that utilizes a series of phases to incorporate into your lifestyle and mindset that may be used to improve wellness.

We all have an opportunity to utilize self-care and awakening to help deal with things like depression and other mental illness. I have, many times, referred to an acronym I read once: C.R.E.A.M—Consciousness Rules Everything Around Me. It's part of the idea that we draw conclusions, right or wrong, from what we observe or are influenced by in our lives. If it's common sense to train our mind to focus on the positives and make it habit, then why are we not all doing it? It's also part of the idea that cognitive tools are often enough to remedy depression and other mental illnesses. Drugs should be a last resort.

Before we continue, I should tell you that my specialty is guiding people to experience the root meaning and cause of the problem(s) they are facing and to bring inner healing to the root emotions involved. My passions are focused listening, helping people with anxiety, and offering support and guidance in a loving and nurturing way. I also support women's health and act as a mental health coach to help those who are suffering with low energy, tiredness, etc.

Think about the metaphor of "moon phases." The idea is that we go through phases just as the moon does. Thinking of life in phases can help us to stay on track without feeling overwhelmed. For example:

- New Moon: this is a time to set intentions, choose new beginnings, embark upon new adventures and make positive changes

- Waxing Moon: now focus on growth, learning, creativity, healing and transformation

- Full Moon: complete the achievement of your goals, harvest what you have sown and protect what you have; it's also a time to focus on cleansing

- Waning Moon: open up, release and let go

Refer to and use the moon phases in your life to consistently reflect on the following ten steps to self-care: After all, the moon is a steady reminder that is always present and looking down on you from the heavens every night. Associating the moon phases to these ten steps is a roadmap to wellness and healthy living.

DRUGS

If you are someone who is troubled by drug use, the moon phase analogy can definitely help you. Before getting into the moon phase analogy here's a little background.

Misuse of prescription drugs is defined as the taking of a medication in a manner or dose other than prescribed; taking someone else's prescription, even if for a legitimate medical complaint such as pain; or taking a medication to feel euphoria (i.e., to get high). The term nonmedical use of prescription drugs also refers to these categories of misuse.

The three classes of medication most commonly misused are:

- opioids—usually prescribed to treat pain

- central nervous system [CNS] depressants—used to treat anxiety and sleep disorders

- stimulants—most often prescribed to treat attention-deficit hyperactivity disorder (ADHD)

Prescription drug misuse can have serious medical consequences. Increases in prescription drug misuse over the last two decades are reflected in increased emergency room visits, overdose deaths associated with prescription drugs, and treatment admissions for prescription drug use disorders, the most severe form of which is addiction. The percentages of prescription abusers seeking medical help is estimated to be in the double digits. Unintentional overdose deaths involving opioid pain relievers have more than quadrupled since 1999 and have long outnumbered those involving heroin and cocaine.

Now if you incorporate the moon phase analogy:

New Moon: make positive changes. First step is a desire to change. You need to believe you are at risk of jeopardizing your own wellbeing if you continue on this path. You need to believe there is a solution and a way out. If you could have done it on your own, chances are you would have done it already. Seek professional counseling. Find a branch of Narcotics Anonymous (designed with the same model as Alcoholics Anonymous), do whatever you can to reduce and eventually end your drug use. Change your focus. Look to substitutes for non-medicinal healthy substitutes to get you that high. Get high on life: it's the quintessential end, isn't it? What we're all searching for? If you aren't happy, look for the reasons why, jot them down, write what needs to change, set a plan to achieve it and, most importantly, work at it tirelessly. Make work and effort the substitute for the high. Bottom line... only YOU can do something about it.

Focus on growth, which is the Waxing Moon. There are many ways to overcome the negatives in life. A psychologist or psychiatrist can offer up cognitive tools or you can try some of the following:

a) Turn your back on darkness or negativity and look to the light. This can mean different things for different people, but the idea is to drive the darkness away, as dark cannot exist where there is light. Personally, I am always looking for the beauty in life. It gives me great joy. I find this beauty in nature, in art, and in the people I meet. I also have the good fortune of having the light of the Lord with me each day. The trick is to look wherever you can find something to lighten your mind and push away dark thoughts that can drag you down into self-abuse.

b) Consciously choose your thoughts and emotions. Life has no meaning unless we put it there. You have the free will to choose to think and feel what you want, no matter what is happening in your life. It's a simple choice that gives you great power. Choose yes or no, forward or backward, up or down, left or right, this thought versus that thought. Whatever the situation is, you can always boil it down to a single choice like good versus bad or light versus dark.

c) Emotion is a wild horse you must learn to tame and ride. Whenever any overwhelming emotion visits you, ring it in and ride it out. Sooner or later it will run out of steam and you will regain control. This kind of focus will take your mind off whatever actions you may have been contemplating when fueled by emotion. This approach will put you in idle mode while you take the wild ride on the stallion of your emotion. It's a safe way to deal with emotions that have the potential to harm. Emotions drive our actions, giving us the impetus to turn our thoughts into behaviours. Better to calm the wild horse and act calmly yourself than let it loose to wreak havoc in your life.

Harvest your efforts (Full Moon). Make sure you take the time to reflect over the past weeks and months to assess and identify where and how you've grown or changed. Celebrate these victories and record what has worked and what hasn't worked. Leap forward and complete some of the goals you have set. Now you'll have even more to celebrate. Reward yourself. Each of us has their own personal idea of what constitutes a reward. You may go out for a nice dinner, take a mini-vacation, or buy that book or movie you've wanted. It could be something as simple as stop for an ice cream cone. You are limited only by your imagination.

Waning Moon: open up, release, let go. Remember that even though you determine the right choice once, you may have to recommit to that same choice numerous times. It takes time to overcome habits and beliefs. The key to developing the long-term behaviours that are necessary for your success is to open up and let go of the old behaviours. You don't need them anymore, so dig them up and show them the light of day. Begin to understand that you are the source of all your thoughts, emotions and actions, and that this gives you complete control—if you are willing to take it. Remember that the drug behaviours are just that: they are behaviours you are choosing, not things that are happening to you. You can just as easily choose a better behaviour in this moment, in the next moment and so on. Eventually you will break the addiction—I guarantee it.

For personal assistance through mental health coaching, please contact **me@wilmadavidaguila.com**.

THE STRUGGLE IS REAL

Don't get me wrong. The struggle people with mental or physical issues have is very real and often requires the help of prescription drugs. The purpose of this chapter is not to deal with the current level of non-medical use of prescription drugs. Instead, I'm directing my words to those who are misusing legitimate prescriptions. These could be people who believe they are sick when what they really need is to learn some tough life skills, or those who began using for legitimate reasons but are now using for the sake of using. None of you deserve to have the small deviations from the set course translate into the huge monkey on your back. What is required is the offer of nonjudgmental help to learn how to deal with the underlying issues that have gotten you to the point where you are now. Psychiatrists, psychologists and some social workers can offer cognitive tools and other life skills to deal with what has, up until now, been dealt with by the misuse of prescription drugs.

The New Moon is a wonderful time to set new goals and make positive changes. To be a useful tool, goal setting must follow a set pattern:

1. The goal must be specific. Not "I am going to stop using drugs," but "I am going to stop using morphine within 30 days, beginning tomorrow morning and with the help of my doctor."

2. The goal must be timely. There's no point in setting a goal for three months from now. It needs to be something you can accomplish today. That's why you always hear about people breaking goals down into "baby steps" or "little bites." A goal is attainable by taking a certain pathway and then making constant course corrections to make sure you stay on that pathway. If a plane or a boat didn't use this same method, they would never reach their desired destination—because small deviations can take them many hundreds of miles off course. So ... take on your goal by making many small decisions and actions designed to get you where you ultimately wish to be, today.

3. You must take massive action. Reverse engineer your goals into their smallest achievable tasks, then act upon them with great vigour. Take the shotgun approach: one shot covers a larger area so as to improve the odds of hitting your target. You can do the same thing. Take as many different actions as you can think of to achieve the goal at hand. Then do the same for the next and the next, until you get to where you want to be.

4. A goal should be something you're passionate about achieving. You can't get anywhere on an empty gas tank. Neither can you achieve a goal if you are emotionally bereft. Emotions tend to move us to action, especially if they are supportive or positive in nature.

The Waxing Moon is a time for focusing on healing, growth and transformation. The very act of setting and achieving goals will teach you and bring you growth. But it is up to you to use the things you learn so as to promote healing and, ultimately, transformation. You must actively focus on change. Why? People just naturally harbour change. It's in our DNA, going back to times when change meant injury or death. The problem is that, today, most change is not injurious. Change is actually beneficial in many ways, and embracing it often uncovers opportunities you might never have otherwise imagined. Focus on transformation. It's a good thing.

The Full Moon is marked by the harvesting of your efforts, the achievement of your big goals. Now is a good time to look at ways of protecting what you've achieved. It's also a time for you to wash away the cobwebs and begin choosing new goals. After all, if you're not moving forward, you're stagnating or even losing ground. If you're not growing you're decaying.

The Waning Moon is marked by the opening up of your mind to the new possibilities represented by the goals you've just set. You can release all responsibility about the decisions you've been thinking about. Now is the time to begin to move forward once again, drawing upon positive emotions only, and letting go of everything else.

I'm a great listener. For personal assistance through coaching, please contact **me@wilmadavidaguila.com**.

MENTAL ATTITUDE

Mental attitude is everything. How can I say this? Well, science has shown that the mind cannot tell the difference between what is clearly imagined and what is real. This is the reason why memory is subjective. It's also the reason why two people who have had the exact same experience may produce conflicting reports about the experience. What does this have to do with drug abuse? Using the concept just described, you can actually imagine yourself well! You see, whatever the mind of man can conceive, it can achieve. No truer statement was ever uttered. If you can see a thing in your mind, like a clear photograph, then you can achieve it. Your mind can't tell that it isn't real. Therefore, when you tell it to attain that clear picture, it will take you out into the world to find or create it.

New Moon: set that intention. Use questions like, "Can you build this for me?" When you get a "Yes," tell your mind to do it, to make it happen. It will listen and obey.

Waxing Moon: use your mind to transform the world and your life. Build something that never existed before you came along, or build a better mousetrap. Your mind is your secret ally.

Full Moon: Take what you have managed to do and protect it to the best of your ability, then rest and prepare to begin anew.

Waning Moon: Let your mind soar. Envision the possibilities as clearly as you possibly can. Prepare for taking new actions.

The topic of mental attitude also relates to one of the most important laws of the universe, the Law of Attraction. This law explains the impact of mental attitude. The Law of Attraction states that we will attract into our lives whatever we are focusing on. It is easy to be unaware of the impact it can have on our lives. Either knowingly or unknowingly, a person sends out thoughts and emotions and attracts back like a magnet more of what they have put out. If you leave your thoughts, emotions and actions unchecked it is easy to attract unwanted things in your life. However, there is also great potential locked within you, and if you apply the Law of Attraction in your life you can encourage the universe to give you great things.

One of the worst parts of misusing drugs is that the artificial feeling you can get from them encourages you to want to use them again to get the relief they give. This signals to the universe that you need more of the drug(s), and that is what the universe will return to you. The same occurs with misinterpreting medical health problems. The more you think you have a health issue, the more the universe tells you that you do. The opposite happens if you believe you can get better, or that you can stop using drugs. The universe will send positive signs, and as your health and lack of dependency improves you will receive more and more benefit from the universe. Focusing on your drug dependency brings more dependency, but focusing on the good in your life brings more good.

When you start sending the right signals into the universe, you have started the New Moon phase. Set your new intentions and welcome positive change. It is a new beginning. As the universe starts to return what you have requested due to the Law of Attraction, the Waxing Moon is in phase and the transformation begins. As your wishes and goals become true, you have harvested what the Law of Attraction and the universe have given you, and the phase reaches a Full Moon. Next the Waning Moon is upon you, and you let go, open up and think of the next thing you want to attract from the universe.

I can help you create more useful attitudes. For personal assistance through coaching, please contact **me@wilmadavidaguila.com**.

REACTIONS

Misinterpreted health issues and the drugs that follow rarely occur spontaneously. They are generally a reaction to something else. To get to the root of this you must inspect your life and find what is root of the reaction(s) that has led you to where you are. What is the stressor that is making you feel health affects and/or leading you to turn to self-medication?

Stress is an inevitable part of life, and completely normal. However, left unchecked it can wreak havoc on your life and happiness. It may arise from something as simple as traffic, an important meeting, or increased work load at the office. It can also be severe and prolonged, such as the stress experienced by those who have faced or still face emotional or physical abuse. When overwhelmed by stress, you may feel defeated, and this inability to cope may lead you to turn to unhealthy solutions such as drug abuse.

Not only is stress troubling in itself, but it can have real physical effects on your body. Physical symptoms can be vast, and commonly include increased heart rate, nausea, dizziness and digestive problems. What you thought had been ailing you may not be the physical illness you found in a book or on the internet, but actually a result of unchecked stress in your life. You may be surprised that some of the physical symptoms you face are healed by simply finding and resolving the source of your stress.

Deciding to find what causes your reactions is a huge first step in overcoming the issues you face. In the New Moon phase, you need to decide to make positive changes in your life. Your intention needs to be focused on finding out the cause of your problems and channeling your reactions in a beneficial way. During the Waxing Moon phase, you will grow and learn about yourself. Once you have identified what causes your reactions, you can transform those reactions into ones that heal you instead of just hiding your problems. As you feel the cleansing effect of constructive reactions you can begin to heal, and during this period you will be under the phase of the Full Moon. You will soon be able to open up, let go and release the baggage of your negative reaction (the Waning Moon).

For personal assistance through coaching, please contact **me@wilmadavidaguila.com**.

AFTERTASTE

When you first turn to drug misuse to solve your problems, they seem sweet. They appear to help you. You might even feel that your life has improved. What you will soon notice, though, is that drugs do not come without a bitter aftertaste. Focusing on this aftertaste is something you can use to motivate yourself to stop drugs and improve your life.

The New Moon phase is the perfect time to recognize the bitter aftertaste drug misuse leaves in your life. It is a time to learn that the drug may not be helping you as much as it seems, and may actually be bringing negativity into your life. It is the time to start on the journey of truly measuring the cons of your use.

As you learn more about the aftertaste of drug misuse, you enter the phase of the Waxing Moon. Your perception starts to grow and your view transforms from only seeing the positives of the drug to understanding that it also introduces negatives. This is an important step in the healing process.

At some point you will realize the drug misuse is just not worth it. This is the phase of the Full Moon. It is a cleansing experience, and the point where you see the drug for the burden that it is. As the Waning Moon phase begins, you let go of your dependency on the drug and open yourself up to a life free of the drugs influence.

I can help you beat your drug problem. Please contact **me@wilmadavidaguila.com**.

COPING

When someone is no longer able to cope with the stresses of life, they begin to look elsewhere for crutches to help keep up, or reasons to explain their failure to cope. Untreated chronic stress can lead to serious health conditions. These conditions include anxiety, insomnia, muscle pain, high blood pressure and a weakened immune system. This explains why some people improperly self-diagnose medical issues and turn to drugs for self-medication. It is important to realize when you begin to no longer be able to keep up and cope with life issues. Learning to cope with stress in healthy ways is an important aspect of a successful life.

Learning to manage stress in a healthy way, when it occurs, can mitigate many of the negative health effects it can cause. People are diverse and different and, thus, so are the ways they can deal with stress. Some people enjoy pursuing hobbies such as team sports, music and art, while others enjoy more solitary activities like meditation, walking and yoga.

I've listed below five healing techniques to help reduce both short and long term success...

1. Take a break from the stressor

It may seem difficult to step away from things like an important work project or a sick child, but when you allow yourself to do so there are many benefits. By giving yourself permission to have space from your stressor you gain the opportunity to do something else, and this in turn allows you to have a new perspective and practice techniques which make you feel less overwhelmed. This doesn't mean avoiding your stress completely, but even a twenty-minute break to take care of yourself can be extremely helpful.

2. Exercise

Everyday more and more research shows that exercise benefits not just the body but also the mind. While most of us know the long-term benefits of exercise, there are also short-term benefits. A quick 20-minute workout or physical activity during a stressful time can rejuvenate you, and improve your focus. This effect is almost immediate and can last for several hours.

3. Smile and laugh

Your emotions and facial expression can send feedback to the brain and have a direct effect on its function. When we are stressed we often hold much of this stress in our faces. Smiling and laughing is an effective way to relieve some of this tension and can improve the situation by signalling to your brain things are not so bad after all.

4. Get social support

If you feel overwhelmed, do not forget you can always call a friend or send someone you trust an email. Sharing your concerns with another person can help relieve your stress. However, trust is important, and you need to know the person will understand and can validate you. If your family is a stressor it may not help to share your work woes with them, and you may be better off calling a close friend.

5. Meditate

One of the best ways to help the mind and body focus and relax is to practice meditation or mindful prayer. The mindfulness that arises from this is a powerful tool to help you see new perspectives, and develop self-compassion and forgiveness. The process allows you to release emotion which may have been causing your body to experience physical stress. Just like exercise research has shown to relieve stress, a brief period of meditation can bring immediate benefits.

The moon phase can help you tackle stress effectively. Identify your stressor and plan how to relieve your stress. This can be thought of as the phase of the New Moon. As you implement your coping mechanisms and your stress begins to release, you are under the Waxing Moon. The Full Moon will signal you can cope with the stressor, and you can face and complete the tasks causing you stress under the Waning Moon without fear.

For coaching in coping and lifestyle skills, please contact **me@wilmadavidaguila.com**.

SIDE EFFECTS

One of the biggest issues with self-diagnosis and drug misuse is that people often only target the side effect. As mentioned before, stress can cause physical problems. Dealing with the physical problems may work temporarily, but the original issues remain. While drugs may make you feel okay, the true problem may still be growing under that shroud you have created, waiting for the right opportunity to reappear and wreak havoc on your life.

Don't assume the issues you face are the only problem. The New Moon is the phase of your life to search for things that may be causing the problems you face. Instead of tackling multiple problems individually and ending up leaving the root cause not dealt with, attack the issue at its source and deal with all the side effects simultaneously. Is your lack of sleep due to a medical issue or is it from the stress of taking on too much at work?

During the Waxing Moon you will discover the truth about your issues, you can learn about how the problems you face arose, and you can begin to heal yourself of your issues. Taking the previous example, you may choose to delegate some of the work. Your sleep might start to improve and you may notice you no longer need those sleeping pills. Additionally, you may see other side effects that you may have missed or linked to another problem. Now that you are not so tired you find yourself helping with the cleaning (for example) and causing less conflict with your spouse. These effects will leave you harvesting the benefits of the Full Moon. Once these side effects have stabilized you will experience the Waning Moon, and can open yourself up to new challenges and let go of the problems of your past.

For someone to listen and to coach you through your stress issues, please contact **me@wilmadavidaguila.com**.

METAPHYSICAL

Drug misuse isn't only related to physical issues but is deeply connected to the metaphysical nature of a person's being. Drug use can be looked at through a spiritual lens. Spirituality refers to belief in a power greater that oneself. One which governs the universe and has a sense of interconnectedness with all living things. It may also involve a quest for self-knowledge, meaning and purpose in one's life. Using drugs is a way to detach and disconnect from the present moment, and all the uncomfortable feelings that go with it. Drug misuse and addiction can also be thought of as having an isolating effect, one that can arise from a lack of connection to one's authentic self, a higher power or persons in the larger community.

Approaching the problems of drug misuse from a spiritual and metaphysical standpoint can be very effective.

One way to approach this is a metaphysical take on the 12 steps, from Ester Nicholson's book *Soul Recovery: The 12 Keys to Healing Addiction*:

1. You are the Power: Through my conscious union with the infinite universal presence, I am powerful, clear and free. Through the realization that God is within me, expressing as me, my life is in divine and perfect order.

2. Restored to wholeness: Through my conscious connection with the one power, I reclaim my spiritual dominion and emotional balance. I am restored to my original nature of clarity, peace and wholeness. I am restored.

3. Complete surrender: I turn my life over to the care of the God I understand, know and embody as love, harmony, peace, health, prosperity and joy. I know that which I am surrendering to, and I do so absolutely. Knowing that this power is the very essence of my being, I say with my whole heart and mind: Thy will be done.

4. An examined life: Through my absolute surrender and conscious connection to the one power and presence, I courageously, deeply and gently search within myself for all thought patterns and behaviours that are out of alignment with love, integrity, harmony and order.

5. Living out loud: I claim the courage and willingness to share the exact nature of my mistakes with another spiritual being. I am heard with compassion, unconditional love and wisdom. In this loving vibration, clarity, peace and balance are restored.

6. Honouring the inner child: I am now ready to release all thought patterns and behaviors unlike my true nature, which is wholeness. I free-fall into the loving presence of spirit within, and allow it to heal

every known and unknown false belief. I am transformed by the renewal of my mind.

7. Never give up: In loving compassion for every aspect of my being, I humbly surrender to the love of spirit. I know myself as a perfect expression of life. I surrender all, and I am restored to the life I am created to live.

8. Willingness: I acknowledge the people I have offended based on false beliefs, fear, doubt and unworthiness. I am willing to go to any lengths to clean up my side of the street.

9. Cleaning up the wreckage: Backed by all the power of the universe, I lovingly, directly and honestly make amends in a way that supports the highest good of all concerned.

10. Spiritual maintenance: I am in tune with my inner self. With integrity, love and self-compassion, I acknowledge my mistakes and continue to clean up the mistakes of my past and present.

11. Conscious contact: Through daily prayer and meditation, I deepen my conscious connection to the divine and experience the fullness of the universal presence as the dynamic reality of my life.

12. Loving service: Through my awakened consciousness, I am now prepared to carry the message of truth out into the world. I am now a clear channel to support the awakening of others to their true identity of wholeness.

The 12 keys or steps also span the phases of the moon. Steps one to four represent the New Moon. Steps five to eight represent the Waxing Moon. Steps nine to 11 represent the Full Moon. And the last step, 12, represents the Waxing Moon.

For spiritual and metaphysical coaching, please contact **me@wilmadavidaguila.com**.

VIBRATION

Vibration is your energetic resonance, and it represents how you think, feel and act. It is the energy the attracts every experience in your life. To ensure happiness and attract good things in your life you want to have positive vibrations. Keeping your vibrations positive will attract positive thoughts and in turn create positive experiences that will match the vibrations of health and abundance. Being in this state is a requirement to attract that which you want.

Dark energies and entities will weaken you and lower your vibrations. Drugs may be a choice you make to try to remedy the state you feel yourself falling into. Drug misuse may trick you into thinking you are improving but actually can bring your vibrations even lower and make a positive state even harder to achieve. Instead of drug misuse you should look into ways to raise your vibration and attract positive energy.

I've included ten steps that can help you raise your vibrations and move away from the vibration lowering temptation of drug misuse:

1. When situations or people drag you down, distance yourself from them so your vibrations are not affected by the negative energy.

2. Raise your energy and awareness by refocusing through daily meditation.

3. A warm bath with Epsom salts and a couple drops of essential oils can help you grow your vibrational energy.

4. Deep breathing is a good way to bring oxygen to your brain and blood stream, and allow your energy to resonate in a positive fashion.

5. Avoid the polluting effect of the toxins from unnecessary drugs, alcohol and nicotine.

6. Find ways to exercise creativity through things like art, poetry, writing or photography.

7. Say what you are grateful for out loud to help grow those vibrations.

8. Be kind to others in your daily activities, and genuinely smile to attract more of the positive energy that comes from it.

9. Exercising at least once a day can deplete negative energy and build positive vibrations.

10. Keeping hydrated keeps your body running efficiently and allows your vibrational level to stay stable.

In the New Moon stage, you need to focus on positive energy and the state of your vibrations. The Waxing Moon is where you will grow your vibrations by focusing on your health and creative outlets. As your vibrations grow you will transition into the Full Moon period and you will feel healing energy, and may even notice transformations beginning in your life. The benefits will start to become apparent as your new vibrational state stabilizes. This signifies the New Moon phase, and many new opportunities will become apparent. As you open yourself up to new energies and let go of negative energy in your life during the Waning Moon, you can prepare for bringing your vibrations to even greater levels.

For personal assistance with building up your energy levels, please contact **me@wilmadavidaguila.com**.

AWAKENING

When you begin to put the lessons from all the previous sections together, you will awaken to the idea that your personal issues or health problems are not always served by drugs. This point is the beginning of the overarching New Moon. It may take you many moon cycles to reach this place. As you learn to release all the various problems through past Waning Moons, accept that the issues you face can be fixed as you surrender yourself to the universe and all the good it can bring you. This Waxing Moon will bring immense growth and overall healing. You will transform into the best version your current self has experienced. The Full Moon will cleanse you and your wish for a life free of drug misuse will come true. The next Waning Moon will allow you open yourself up to all the potential that was already there but that you had not been able to see.

For personal assistance through coaching or for group seminars, please contact **me@wilmadavidaguila.com**.

Step Into Greatness

LES BROWN

Y ou have greatness within you. You can do more than you could ever imagine. The problem most people have is that they set a goal and then ask "how can I do it? I don't have the necessary skills or education or experience".

I know what that's like. I wasted 14 years on asking myself how I could be a motivational speaker. My mind focused on the negative—on the things that were in my way, rather than on the things that were not.

It's not what you don't have but what you think you need that keeps you from getting what you want from life. But, when the dream is big enough, the obstacles don't matter. You'll get there if you stay the course. Nothing can stop you but death itself.

Think about that last statement for a minute. There's nothing on this earth that can stop you from achieving what it is that you want. So, get out of your way, and quit sabotaging your dreams. Do everything in your power to make them happen—because you cannot fail!

They say the best way to die is with your loved ones gathered around your bed. But what if you were dying and it was the ideas you never acted upon, the gifts you never used and the dreams you never pursued, that were circled around your bed? Answer that question right now. Write down your answers. If you die this very moment what ideas, what gifts, what dreams will die with you?

Then say: I refuse to die an unlived life! You beat out 40 million sperm to get here, and you'll never have to face such odds again. Walk through the field of life and leave a trail behind.

One day, one of my rich friends brought my mother a new pair of shoes for me. Now, even though we weren't well off, I didn't want them; they were a size nine and I was a size nine and a half. My mother didn't listen and told my sister to go get some Vaseline, which she rubbed all over my feet. Then my mother had me put those shoes on, minding that I didn't scrunch down the heel. She had my sister run some water in the bathtub, and I was told to get in and walk around in the water. I said that my feet hurt. She just ignored me and asked about my day at school, how everything went and did I get into any fights? I knew what she was up to, that she was trying to distract me, so I said I had only gotten into three fights. After a while mother asked me if my feet still hurt. I admitted that the pain had indeed lessened. She kept me walking in that tub until I had a brand new pair of comfortable, size nine and a half shoes.

You see, once the leather in the shoes got wet, they stretched! And what you need to do is stretch a little. I believe that most people don't set high goals and miss them, but rather, they set lower goals and hit them and then they stay there, stuck on the side of the highway of life. When you're pursuing your greatness, you don't know what your limitations are, and you need to act like you don't have any. If you shoot for the moon and miss, you'll still be in the stars.

You also need coaching (a mentor). Why? There are times you, too, will find yourself parked on the side of the highway of life with no gas in the vehicle. What you need then is someone to stop and offer to pick up some gas down the road a ways and bring it back to you. That person is your coach. Yes, they are there for advice, but their main job is to help you through the difficulties that life throws at all of us.

Another reason for having a coach is that you can't see the picture when you're in the frame. In other words, he or she can often see where you are with a clarity and focus that's unavailable to you. They're not going to leave you parked along the road of life, nor are they going to allow you to be stuck in the moment like a photo in a frame.

And let's say you just can't see your way forward. You don't believe it's possible. Sometimes you just have to believe in someone's belief in you. This could be your coach, a loved one or even a staunch friend. You need to hear them say you can do it, time and again. Because, after all, faith comes from hearing and hearing and hearing.

Look at it this way. Most people fail because of possibility blindness. They can't see what lies before them. There are always possibilities. Because of this, your dream is possible. You may fail often. In fact, I want you to say this: I will fail my way to success. Here is why.

I had a TV show that failed. I felt I had to go back to public speaking. I had failed, so I parked my car for ten years. Then I saw Dr. Wayne Dyer was still on PBS and I decided to call them. They said they would love to work with me and asked where I had been. I wasn't as good as I had been ten years before, as I was out of practice, but I still had to get back in the game. I was determined to drive on empty.

Listen to recordings, go to seminars, challenge yourself, and you'll begin to step into your greatness, you'll begin to fill yourself with the energy you need to climb to greater heights. Most people never attend a seminar. They won't invest money in books or audio programs. You put yourself in the top 5 percent just by making a different choice than the average person. This is called contrary thinking. It's a concept taken from the financial industry. One considers choosing the exact opposite behaviour of the average person as a way to get better than average results. You don't have to make the contrarian choice, but if you don't have anything to lose by going that road, why not consider the option?

Make your move before you're ready. Walk by faith not by sight and make sure you're happy doing it. If you can't be happy, what else is there? Helen Keller said, "Life is short, eat the dessert first."

What is faith? Many of us think of God when we think of faith. A different viewpoint claims that faith is a firm belief in something for which there is no proof. I would rather think of faith as something that is believed especially with strong conviction. It is this last definition I am referring to when I say walk by faith not by sight. Be happy and go forth with strong conviction that you are destined for greatness.

An important step on your way to greatness is to take the time to detoxify. You've got to look at the people in your life. What are they doing for you? Are they setting a pace that you can follow? If not, whose pace have you adjusted to? If you're the smartest in your group, find a new group.

Are the people in your life pulling you down or lifting you up? You know what to do, right? Banish the negative and stay with the positive; it's that simple. Dr. Norman Vincent Peale once said (when I was in the audience), "You are special. You have greatness within you, and you can do more than you could ever possibly imagine."

He overrode the inner conversations in my mind and reached the heart of me. He set me on fire. This is yet another reason for seeking out the help of a coach or mentor or other new people in your life. They can do what Dr. Peale did for me. They can set your passion free.

How important is it to have the right kind of person/people on your side? There was a study done that determined it takes 16 people saying you can do something to overcome one person who says you can't do something. That's right, one negative, unsupportive person can wipe out the work of 16 other supportive people. The message can't be any clearer than that.

Let's face the cold, hard truth: most people stay in park along the highway of life. They never feel the passion, the love for their fellow man, or for the work they do. They are stuck in the proverbial rut. What's the reason? There are many reasons, but only one common factor: fear — fear of change, fear of failure, fear of success, fear they may not be good enough, fear of competition, even fear of rejection.

"Rejection is a myth," says Jack Canfield, co-author of The Chicken Soup for the Soul series. "It's not like you get a slap in the face each time you are rejected." Why not take every "no" you receive as a vitamin, and every time you take one know you are another step closer to success.

You will win if you don't quit. Even a broken clock is right twice a day.

Professional baseball players, on average, get on base just three times out of every ten times they face the opposing pitcher. Even superstars fail half of the time they appear at the plate.

Top commissioned salespeople face similar odds. They make may make one sale from every three people they see, but it will have taken them between 75 and 100 telephone calls to make the 15 appointments they need to close their five sales for the week. And these are statistics for the elite. Most salespeople never reach these kinds of numbers.

People don't spend their lives working for just one company anymore. This means you must build up a set of skills and experiences that are portable. This can be done a number of ways, but my favourite approaches follow.

You must be willing to do the things others won't do in order to have tomorrow the things that others don't have. Provide more service than you get paid for. Set some high standards for yourself.

Begin each day with your most difficult task. The rest of the day will seem more enjoyable and a whole lot easier.

Someone needs help with a problem? Be the solution to that problem.

Also, find those tasks that are being consistently ignored and do them. You'll be surprised by the results. An acquaintance of mine used this approach at a number of entry-level positions and each time he quickly ended up being offered a position in management.

You must increase your energy. Kick it up a notch. We are spirits having a physical existence; let your spirit shine. Quit frittering away your energy. Use it to move you closer to the achievement of your dreams. Refuse to spend it on non-productive activities.

What do people say about you when you leave a room? Are you willing to take responsibility—to walk your talk. There is a terrible epidemic sweeping our nation, and it is the refusal to take responsibility for one's actions. Consider that at some point in any situation there will have been a moment where you could have done something to change the outcome. To that end you are responsible for what happened. It's a hard thing to accept, but it's true.

Life's hard. It was hard when I was told I had cancer. I had sunken into despair, and was hiding away in my study when my son came in. My son asked me if I was going to die. What could I do? I told him I was going to fight, even though I was scared. I also told him that I needed some help. Not because I was weak but because I wanted to stay strong. Keep asking until you get help. Don't stop until you get it.

A setback is the setup for a comeback. A setback is simply a misstep on the long road of success. It means nothing in the larger scheme of things. And, surprisingly, it sets you up for your next win. It tends to focus you and your energy on your immediate goals, paving the way for your next sprint, for your comeback.

It's worth it. Your dreams are worth the sacrifices you'll have to make to achieve them. Find five reasons that will make your dreams worth it for you. Say to yourself, I refuse to live an unlived life.

If you are casual about your dreams, you'll end up a casualty. You must be passionate about your dreams, living and breathing them throughout your days. You've got to be hungry! People who are hungry refuse to take no for an answer. Make NO your vitamin. Be unstoppable. Be hungry.

Let me give you an example of what I mean by hungry …

I decided I wanted to become a disc jockey, so I went down to the local radio station and asked the manager, Mr. Milton "Butterball" Smith, if he had a job available for a disc jockey. He said he did not. The next day I went back, and Mr. Smith asked "Weren't you here yesterday?" I explained that I was just checking to see if anyone was sick or had died. He responded by telling me not to come back again. Day three, I went back again—with the same story. Mr. Smith told me to get out of there. I came back the fourth day and gave Mr. Smith my story one more time. He was so beside himself that he told me to get him a cup of coffee. I said, "Yes, sir!" That's how I became the errand boy.

While working as an errand boy at the station, I took every opportunity to hang out with the deejays and to observe them working. After I had taught myself how to run the control room, it was just a matter of biding my time.

Then one day an opportunity presented itself. One of the disc jockeys by the name of Rockin' Roger was drinking heavily while he was on the air. It was a Saturday afternoon. And there I was, the only one there.

I watched him through the control-room window. I walked back and forth in front of that window like a cat watching a mouse, saying "Drink, Rock, Drink!" I was young. I was ready. And I was hungry.

Pretty soon, the phone rang. It was the station manager. He said, "Les, this is Mr. Klein."

I said, "Yes, I know."

He said, "Rock can't finish his program."

I said, "Yes sir, I know."

He said, "Would you call one of the other disc jockeys to fill in?"

I said, "Yes sir, I sure will, sir."

And when he hung up, I said, "Now he must think I'm crazy." I called up my mama and my girlfriend, Cassandra, and I told them, "Ya'll go out on the front porch and turn up the radio, I'M ABOUT TO COME ON THE AIR!"

I waited 15 or 20 minutes and called the station manager back. I said, "Mr. Klein, I can't find NOBODY!"

He said, "Young boy, do you know how to work the controls?"

I said, "Yes, sir."

He said, "Go in there, but don't say anything. Hear me?"

I said, "Yes, sir."

I couldn't wait to get old Rock out of the way. I went in there, took my seat behind that turntable, flipped on the microphone and let 'er rip.

"Look out, this is me, LB., triple P. Les Brown your platter-playin' papa. There were none before me and there will be none after me, therefore that makes me the one and only. Young and single and love to mingle, certified, bona fide and indubitably qualified to bring you satisfaction and a whole lot of action. Look out baby, I'm your LOVE man."

I WAS HUNGRY!

During my adult life I've been a deejay, a radio station manager, a Democrat in the Ohio Legislature, a minister, a TV personality, an author and a public speaker, but I've always looked after what I valued most—my mother. What I want for her is one of my dreams, one of my goals.

My life has been a true testament to the power of positive thinking and the infinite human potential. I was born in an abandoned building on a floor in Liberty City, a low-income section of Miami, Florida, and adopted at six weeks of age by Mrs. Mamie Brown, a 38-year-old single woman, cafeteria cook and domestic worker. She had very little education or financial means, but a very big heart and the desire to care for myself and my twin brother. I call myself Mrs. Mamie Brown's Baby Boy and I say that all that I am and all that I ever hoped to be, I owe to my mother.

My determination and persistence in searching for ways to help my mother overcome poverty and developing my philosophy to do whatever it takes to achieve success led me to become a distinguished authority on harnessing human potential and success. That philosophy is best expressed by the following ...

"If you want a thing bad enough to go out and fight for it,
to work day and night for it,
to give up your time, your peace and your sleep for it...
if all that you dream and scheme is about it,
and life seems useless and worthless without it...
if you gladly sweat for it and fret for it and plan for it
and lose all your terror of the opposition for it...
if you simply go after that thing you want
with all of your capacity, strength and sagacity,
faith, hope and confidence and stern pertinacity...
if neither cold, poverty, famine, nor gout,
sickness nor pain, of body and brain,
can keep you away from the thing that you want...
if dogged and grim you beseech and beset it,
with the help of God, you will get it!"

Branding Small Business

RAYMOND AARON

B randing is an incredibly important tool for creating and building your business. Large companies have been benefiting from branding ever since people first started selling things to other people. Branding made those businesses big.

If you're a small business owner, you probably imagine that small companies are different and don't need branding as much as large companies do. Not true. The truth is small businesses need branding just as much, if not more, than large companies.

Perhaps you've thought about branding, but assumed you'd need millions of dollars to do it properly, or that branding is just the same thing as marketing. Nothing could be further from the truth.

Marketing is the engine of your company's success. Branding is the fuel in that engine.

In the old days, salespeople were a big part of the selling process. They recommended one product over another and laid out the reasons why it was better. Salespeople had credibility because they knew about all the products, and customers often took the advice they had to offer.

Today, consumers control the buying process. They shop in big box stores, super-sized supermarkets, and over the Internet — where there are no salespeople. Buyers now get online and gather information beforehand. They learn about all the products available and look to see if there really is any difference between them. Consumers also read reviews and check social media to see if both the company and the product are reputable. In other words, they want to know what the brand is all about.

The way of commerce used to be: "Nothing happens till something is sold." Today it's: "Nothing happens till something is branded!"

DEFINING A BRAND

A brand is a proper name that stands for something. It lives in the consumer's mind, has positive or negative characteristics, and invokes a feeling or an image. In short, it's a person's perception of a product or a company.

When all goes well, consumers associate the same characteristics with a brand that the company talks about in its advertising, public relations, marketing and sales materials. Of course, when a product doesn't live up to what the company says about it, the brand gets a bad reputation. On the other hand, if a product or service over-delivers on the promises made, the brand can become a superstar.

RECOGNIZING BRANDING AND ITS CHARACTERISTICS

Branding is the science and art of making something that isn't unique, unique. Branding in the marketplace is the same as branding on a ranch. On a ranch, ranchers use branding to differentiate their cattle from every other rancher's cattle (because all cattle look pretty much the same). In the marketplace, branding is what makes a product stand out in a crowd of similar products. The right branding gets you noticed, remembered and sold — or perhaps I should say bought, because today it is all about buying, not selling.

There are four main characteristics of branding that make it an integral part of the marketing and purchasing process.

1. Branding makes you trustworthy and known

Branding makes a product more special than other products. With branding, a normal, everyday product has a personality, and a first and last name, and people know who you are.

In today's marketplace, most products are, more or less, just like their competition. Toilet paper is toilet paper, milk is milk, and a grocery store by any other name is still a grocery store. However, branding takes a product and makes it unique. For example, high-quality drinking water is available from just about every tap in the Western world and it's free, but people pay good money for it when it comes in a bottle. Branding takes bottled water and makes Evian.

Furthermore, every aspect of your brand gives potential customers a feeling or comfort level that they associate with you. The more powerful and positive that feeling is, the more easily and more frequently they will want to do business with you and, indeed, will do business with you.

2. Branding differentiates you from others

Strong branding makes you better than your competition, and makes your product name memorable and easy to remember. Even if your product is absolutely the same as every other product like it, branding makes it special. Branding makes it the first product a consumer thinks about when deciding to make a purchase.

Branding also makes a product seem popular. Everyone knows about it, which implicitly says people like it. And, if people like it, it must be good.

3. Branding makes you worth more money

The stronger your branding is, the more likely people are willing to spend that little bit extra because they believe you, your product, your service, or your business are worth it. They may say they won't, but they will. They do it all the time.

For example, a one-pound box of Godiva chocolates costs about $40; the same weight of Hershey's Kisses costs about $4. The quality of the chocolate isn't ten times greater. The reason people buy Godiva is that the brand Godiva means "gift" whereas the brand Hershey means "snack". Gifts obviously cost more than snacks.

4. Branding pre-sells your product

In the buying age, people most often make the decision on which products to pick up before they walk into the store. The stronger the branding, the more likely people are to think in terms of your product rather than the product category. For example, people are as likely, maybe even more likely, to add Hellmann's to the shopping list as they are to write down simply mayo. The same is true for soda, ketchup, and many other products with successful, strong branding.

Plus, as soon as a shopper gets to the shelf, branding can provide a quick reminder of what products to grab in a few ways:

- An icon or logo
- A specific color
- An audio icon

BRANDING IN A SMALL BUSINESS

Big companies spend millions of dollars on advertising, marketing, and public relations (PR) to build recognition of a new product name. They get their selling messages out to the public using television, radio, magazines, and the Internet. They can even throw money at damage control when necessary. The strategies for branding are the same in a small business, but the scale, costs, and a few of the tactics change.

Make your brand name work harder

The name of a small business can mean everything in terms of branding. Your brand name needs to work harder for your business than you do. It's the first thing a prospective customer sees, and it is how they will remember you. A brand name has to be memorable when spoken, and focused in its meaning. If the name doesn't represent what consumers believe about a product and the company that makes it, then that brand will fail.

In building your product's reputation and image, less is often significantly more. Make sure the name you choose immediately gives a sense of what you do.

Large corporations have millions of dollars to take a meaningless brand name and make it stand for something. Small businesses don't, so use words that really mean something. Strive for something interesting and be right on point. You don't need to be boring.

Plumbers, for example, would do well setting themselves apart with names like "The On-Time Plumber" or "24/7 Plumbing". The same is true for electricians, IT providers, or even marketing consultants. Plenty of other types of business are so general in nature they just don't work hard enough in a business or product name.

Even the playing field: The Net

The Internet has leveled the playing field for small businesses like nothing else. You can use the Internet in several ways to market your brand:

Website: Developing and maintaining a website is easier than ever. Anyone can find your business regardless of its size.

Social Media: Facebook and Twitter can promote your brand in a cost-effective manner.

BUILDING YOUR BRAND WITH THE BRANDING LADDER

Even if you do everything perfectly the first time (and I don't know anyone who does), branding takes time. How much time isn't just up to you, but you can speed things along by understanding the different levels of branding, as well as the business and marketing strategies that can get you to the top.

Introducing the Branding Ladder

Moving through the levels of branding is like climbing a ladder to the top of the marketplace. The Branding Ladder has five distinct rungs and, unlike stairs, you can't take them two at a time. You have to take them in order, and some businesses spend more time on each rung than others.

You can also think of the Branding Ladder in terms of a scale from zero to ten. Everyone starts at zero. If you properly climb the ladder, you can end up at 12 out of 10. The Branding Ladder below shows a special rung at the top of the ladder that can take your business over the top. The following section explains the Branding Ladder and how your small business can move up it.

THE BRANDING LADDER	
Brand Advocacy	**12/10**
Brand Insistence	**10/10**
Brand Preference	**3/10**
Brand Awareness	**1/10**
Brand Absence	**0/10**

Rung 1: Living in the void

Your business, in fact every business, starts at the bottom rung, which is called brand absence, meaning you have no brand whatsoever except your own name. On a scale of one to ten, brand absence is, of course, zero. That's the worst place to live and obviously the most difficult entrepreneurially. The good news is that the only way is up.

Ninety-seven percent of businesses live on this rung of the Branding Ladder. They earn far less than they want to earn, far less than they should earn, and far less than they would earn if they did exactly the same work under a real brand.

Rung 2: Achieving awareness

Brand awareness is a good first step up the ladder to the second rung. Actually, it's really good, especially because 97 percent of businesses never get there. You want people to be aware of you. When person A speaks to person B and says, "Have you heard of "The 24/7 Plumber?" You want the answer to be "yes".

On that scale of one to ten, however, brand awareness is only a one. It's better than nothing, but not that much better. Although people know of your brand, being aware doesn't mean that they are interested in buying it. Coca Cola drinkers know about Pepsi, but they don't drink it.

Rung 3: Becoming the preferred brand

Getting to the third rung, brand preference, is definitely a real step up. This rung means that people prefer to use your product or service rather than that of your competition. They believe there is a real difference between you and others, and you're their first choice. This rung is a crucial branding stage for parity products, such as bottled water and breakfast cereals, not to mention plumbers, electricians, lawyers, and all the others. Brand preference is clearly better than brand awareness, but it's less than halfway up the ladder.

Car rental companies represent a perfect example of why brand preference may not be enough. When someone lands at an airport and needs to rent a car on the spot, he or she may go straight to the preferred rental counter. If that company has a car available, it's a sale. However, if all the cars for that company have been rented, the person will move to the next rental kiosk without much thought, because one rental car is just as good as another.

Exerting Brand Preference needs to be easy and convenient

If all you have is brand preference, your business is on shaky ground and you can lose business for the feeblest of reasons. Very few people go to a second or third supermarket just to find their favorite brand of bottled water. Similarly, a shopper may prefer one store over another but, if both stores sell the same products, he or she will often go to the closest store even if it is not the better liked one. The reason for staying nearby does not need to be a dramatic one — the shopper may simply be tired, on a tight schedule, or not in the mood to travel.

Rung 4: Making it you and only you

When your customers are so committed to your product or service that they won't accept a substitute, you have reached the fourth rung of the Branding Ladder. All companies strive to reach this place, called brand insistence.

Brand insistence means that someone's experience with a product in terms of performance, durability, customer service, and image has been sufficiently exceptional. As a result, the product has earned an incredible level of loyalty. If the product isn't available where the customer is, he or she will literally not buy something else. Rather, the person will look for the preferred product elsewhere. Can you imagine what a fabulous place this is for a company to be? Brand insistence is the best of the best, the perfect ten out of ten, the whole ball of wax.

Apple is a perfect example of brand insistence

Apple users don't just think, they know in their heads and hearts, that anything made by Apple is technologically-advanced, user-friendly, and just all-around superior. Committed to everything Apple, Mac users won't even entertain the thought that a PC may have positive attributes.

Apple people love everything about their Macs, iPads, iPhones, the Mac stores and all those apps. When the company introduces a new product, many of its brand-insistent fans actually wait in line overnight to be one of the first to have it. Steve Jobs is one of their idols.

Considering one big potential problem

Unfortunately, you can lose brand insistence much more quickly than you can achieve it. Brand-insistent customers have such high expectations that they can be disillusioned or disappointed by just one bad product experience. You also have to consistently reinforce the positives because insistence can fade over time. Even someone who has bought and re-bought a specific brand of car for the last 20 years can decide it's just time for a change. That's how fickle the world is.

At ten out of ten, brand insistence may seem like the top rung of the ladder, but it's not. One rung is actually better, and it involves getting your brand-insistent customers to keep polishing your brand for you.

Rung 5: Getting customers to do the work for you

Brand advocacy is the highest rung on the ladder. It's better than ten out of ten because you have customers who are so happy with your product that they want everyone to know about it and use it. Think of them as uber-fans. Not only do they recommend you to friends and family, they also practically shout your praises from the rooftops, interrupt conversations among strangers to give their opinion, and tell everyone they meet how fantastic you are. Most companies can only aspire to this level of customer satisfaction. Apple is one of the few large corporations in recent history that has brand advocates all over the world.

- Brand advocacy does the following five extraordinary things for your company. Brand advocacy:

- Provides a level of visibility that you couldn't pay for if you tried. Brand advocates are so enthusiastic they talk about you all the time, and reach people in ways general media and public relations can't. You get great visibility because they make sure people actually listen.

- Delivers free advertising and public relations. Companies love the extra super-positive messaging, all for free.

- Affords a level of credibility that literally can't be bought. Brand advocates are more than just walking testimonials. They are living proof that you are the best.

- Provides pre-sold prospective customers. Advocate recommendations carry so much weight that they are worth much more than plain referrals. They deliver customers ready and committed to purchasing your product or service.

- Increases profits exponentially. Brand advocates are money-making machines for your business because they increase sales and decrease marketing costs.

For these reasons, brand advocacy is 12 out of 10!!

BRANDING YOURSELF:
HOW TO DO SO IN FOUR EASY WAYS

If you're interested in branding your product or company, you may not be sure where to begin. The good news: I'm here to help. You can brand in many ways, but here I pare it down to four ways to help you start:

Branding by association

This way involves hanging out with and being seen with people who are very much higher than you in your particular niche.

Branding by achievement

This way repurposes your previous achievements.

Branding by testimonial

This way makes use of the testimonials that you receive but have likely never used.

Branding by WOW

A WOW is the pleasantly unexpected, the equivalent of going the extra mile. The easiest and most certain way to WOW people is to tell them that you've written a book. To discover how you can write a book of own, go to www.BrandingSmallBusinessForDummies.com.

Sex, Love and Relationships

DR. JOHN GRAY

Just as great sex is important to lasting love, good health is important to sex and relationships. About 12 years ago, I cured myself of early stage Parkinson's disease. The doctors were amazed, but my wife was even more amazed. She noted that our relationship and sex life had become dramatically better. It turns out that the natural supplements I used to reverse Parkinson's can also make you more attentive and loving in your relationship. At that point, I realized that good relationship skills alone were not enough to sustain love and passion for a lifetime.

I shared many insights gained from my 40 years' experience as a marriage counselor and coach in *Men Are From Mars, Women Are From Venus*. And while my insights go a long way towards helping men and women understand and support each other, good communication skills alone are not always enough. For better relationships, we not only need to be healthy, but we must also experience optimum brain function.

If you are tired, depressed, anxious, not sleeping well, or in pain, then certainly romantic feelings will become a thing of the past. My recovery from Parkinson's revealed to me the profound connection between the quality of our health and our relationships. This insight has motivated me, over the past twelve years, to research the secrets of optimum health as a foundation for lasting love.

These are health secrets that are generally not explored in medical school. In medical school, doctors are indoctrinated into the culture of examining the symptoms, identifying the sickness, and prescribing a drug to treat that sickness. They learn very little about how to be healthy or to sustain successful relationships.

There are no university courses entitled "Better Nutrition For Better Sex". Drugs sometimes save lives, but they also have negative side effects that do little to preserve the passion in a relationship. Ideally, drugs should be used as a last resort and 90 % of our health plan should be drug free. From this perspective, the heath care crisis, as well as our high rate of divorce in America, is indirectly caused by our dependence on doctors and prescription drugs.

Most people have not even considered that taking prescribed drugs (even for the small stuff) can weaken their relationships, which in turn makes them more vulnerable to more disease. For example, if you are feeling depressed or anxious, a drug may numb your pain, but it does nothing to help you correct the cause of your problem. It can even prevent you from feeling your natural motivation to get the emotional support you need. In a variety of ways, our common health complaints are all expressions of two major conditions: our lack of education to identify and support unmet gender-specific emotional needs; and our lack of education to identify and support unmet gender-specific nutritional needs.

With an understanding of natural solutions that have been around for thousands of years, drugs are not needed to treat many common complaints. Some symptoms like low energy, weight gain, allergies, hormonal imbalance, mood swings, poor sleep, indigestion, lack of focus, ADD and ADHD, procrastination, low motivation, memory loss, decreased libido, PMS, vaginal dryness, muscle and joint pain, or the lack of passion in life and/or our relationships can be treated drug-free. By using drugs (even over-the-counter drugs) to treat these common complaints, our bodies and relationships are weakened, making us more vulnerable to bigger and more costly health challenges like cancer, diabetes, heart disease, auto-immune disease, dementia, and Alzheimer's. In simple terms, by handling the easy stuff (the common complaints) without doctors and drugs, we can protect ourselves from the big stuff (cancer, heart disease, dementia, etc.) We can be healthy and also enjoy lasting love and passion in our personal lives.

Even if you are taking anti-depressants or hormone replacement therapy, sometimes all it takes to stop treating the symptom is to directly handle the cause. With specific mineral orotates (something most people have never heard of) or omega three oil from the brains of salmon, your stress levels immediately drop and you begin to feel happy and in love again.

For every health challenge, we have explored the effects on our relationships, with as well as natural remedies that can sometimes produce immediate positive results. You can find these natural solutions to common health complaints for free at my website: www.MarsVenus.com.

What they don't teach in medical school is how to be healthy and happy without the use of drugs or hormone replacement. By refusing drugs and taking responsibility for your health, a wealth of new possibilities can become available to you. We are designed to be healthy and happy, and it is within our reach if we commit to increasing our knowledge.

New research regarding the brain differences in men and women reveals how specific nutritional supplements, combined with gender-specific relationship and self-nurturing skills, can stimulate the hormones of health, happiness and increased energy. Over the past 10 years in my healing center in California, I witnessed how natural solutions coupled with gender-specific relationship skills could solve our common health complaints without drugs. By addressing these common complaints without prescribed drugs, not only do we feel better, but our relationships have the potential to improve dramatically.

Ultimately the cause of all our common complaints is higher stress levels. Researchers around the world all agree that chronic stress levels in our bodies provide a basis for any and all disease to take hold. An easy and quick solution for lowering our stress reactions is specific nutritional support combined with gender-smart relationship skills. Extra nutritional support is needed because stress depletes the body very quickly of essential nutrients. When a car engine is running more quickly, it uses fuel more quickly. When we are stressed, we need both extra nutrients and extra emotional support. Understanding what we need to take and where to get it requires education. Every week day at www.MarsVenus.com I have a live daily show where I freely answer questions and provide this much-needed new gender-specific insight.

At www.MarsVenus.com, we are happy to share what we have learned for creating healthy bodies and positive relationships. You can find a host of natural solutions for common complaints and feel confident that you have the power to feel fully alive with an abundance of energy and positive feelings that will enrich all your relationships.

Your Life Energy

AMAL INDI

I have 20 years of experience in the tech sector and corporate banking. In my previous life in the "Rat Race", I was waking up every day and going to a job that provided well for me. After some major changes in my life (including a divorce), I started recognizing that I wasn't intrinsically happy. I would be going about my day filled with negative thoughts and emotions. It felt as though they were taking over in a way, and I recognized how they were beginning to affect every moment of my day and every interaction with those around me. I refer to these as "Thought Bugs", which I will go on to explain later. These Thought Bugs were almost like a computer virus, affecting all the thoughts or, as one may say, programming in my mind. After recognizing these Bugs and studying them in myself for many years, I began to draw strong conclusions about how I could create positive change in my mind. This positive change in my thoughts would eventually lead to me leaving the "Rat Race" and starting on the mission of my life to share my new paradigm with those around me. I believe that we can change our minds and create a positive and uplifting life, not only for ourselves, but for those around us. I would love to share with you the basics of what I discovered, a new way of examining our thought patterns and how to drastically shift the energy around you (your Aura) so that you can lead a fantastic life!

GETTING STARTED ON YOUR OWN JOURNEY

When was the last time you really felt 100%? When I say 100%, I mean you wake up feeling a general positivity in your mood, you are looking forward to a new day, your interactions with people feel good, and you walk around feeling a general sense of purpose even with the simple tasks of getting groceries or whatever your work environment. You may think that you have no say in how you really feel. That deep down, you cannot control your thoughts and emotions. I know that this is not true. I developed a unique way of seeing our minds and how deeply they affect our energy. Have you heard of life energy, such as positive energy, negative energy, Aura energy, and universal energy? Read on!

WHAT MAKES US HUMAN?

Each one of us is a biological marvel of different cells, tissues, genes. These are the many working pieces that come together to create our human body. What really makes us human in a whole sense? We each possess an in-depth energetic landscape that we can't deny. This energetic pulse is used by scientists and technicians daily to perform tests and create pictures of our bodies and their functions. Think of the neuroscientists that connect our bodies to electrodes and measure our brain waves. That's part of it. We can't deny there is a part of us beyond just the tissues of our muscles and bones.

Did you know that surrounding you right now is an energy field that is all your own? This energetic field is referred to as your Aura. This Aura can be the beginning of a life that you love. Every human being has an energy field around them. We cannot see this field with the naked eye. However, we can see this field with an Aura machine. It's true! I personally have had mine captured and what was reflected back to me (in terms of energetic levels) was what I was truly feeling.

Your Aura and the energy you radiate is 100% in your control. Some days, you might feel positive and good, while other days, you may feel more negative and lower. These are your energy levels. They can vibrate high or low. It depends on you and your thoughts. Remember, with improvements to your mind and thoughts, your aura energy field will continuously change, thus altering the life you are leading.

YOUR AURA

Over the centuries of humans existing and contemplating our existence, many have acknowledged the fact that we have an energy that extends beyond our skin and flesh, which can actually interact with the world around us. This is referred to as your body's Aura. The Aura refers to the energy around your body that can be affected from the inside out or the outside in. When it is strong, the Aura around your body can extend quite a way beyond the barrier of your physical body (your skin). It can also manifest as different colours, depending on the emotional mood of the person. For example, when you are in a state of calm, then you will exude a white Aura. When you are in a state of anger, then you will exude a red Aura. Sometimes Auras may also be a combination of different colours. There is technology now that can show the colour and strength of someone's Aura. I have had mine checked. One day, it was light in colour and extended far beyond my body. This didn't surprise me as I feel I live in a state of calm, clear energy and my inner emotional landscape is positive. If you were to have an opportunity to get yours checked today what do you think the results would be? Strong and white? Or weak and maybe red? Maybe you feel like it may not show up at all.

This is what I want to teach you. This is my mission right now: To help you understand that you can empower yourself and create a strong, positive Aura that will not only affect your overall sense of well-being. It will affect your relationships, your business, and your life as a whole.

YOUR HUMAN SYSTEM

Through my own exploration, I began seeing and noticing a pattern in how my Aura was being affected by different things in my life. As I continued to study this in myself, it became clear to me that that there were specific things in play, and it was all rooted in my mind. Having a strong background in technology, I began to clearly see how our own minds behave like supercomputers. (Stay with me here!) Just like a super computer, we have our own operating system and the ability to run many programs at once. We are constantly juggling responsibilities, taking in the world around us, assessing how we feel, and determining what we need. The list could go on and on! Just take a moment right now: close your eyes and connect to all the "programs" open in your mind that are constantly running. Relate that to being connected to your own unique operating system of your mind. Now imagine that a computer virus was implanted into one of your programs and began affecting your thoughts. Computer viruses are designed to spread to all parts of a computer with the goal of eventually changing the computer, more often than not, making it completely dysfunctional. This is what can happen in your mind. A negative thought may enter your mind about something specific. Maybe a co-worker engages you in conversation about a rumour that someone is up for raise (one that you applied for) or on your coffee break the barista makes a mistake on your order and you feel it ruins your morning. I call these viruses of our thoughts Human Errors. In its most basic form, Human Errors can be outlined as the following emotions, or what I like to call Thought Bugs:

- Anger
- Suspicion
- Craving
- Comparison
- Low self-esteem
- Procrastination
- Getting stuck in negative thoughts

What it can be boiled down to is that these negative thought bugs can enter into your mind, which in turn creates negative energy. This leads to stress and a weakening of your Aura.

I'm sure you can think of a definitive moment, probably even within the last day or the last week, where you can see how your own errors were affecting your core system and negatively impacting the energy around you.

Luckily, we have a set of more positive emotions and various ways of reacting that counter the negative ones. I have identified these and aptly named them our Human Features.

Primary Human features that combat the errors include:
- Love and kindness
- Acceptance
- Forgiveness
- Courageousness
- Patience
- Authenticity
- Gratefulness

One can think of these features as a built-in tool box to combat negativity. This is always at our disposal! I want to help you identify where these positive emotions are in you, so that you may have access them and strengthen the energy that you are putting out into the world and your Aura.

Look, I am not a psychologist. I am not a therapist. I am, however, a believer in how we show up to our work and interact with those around us will have a deep impact on the life we are creating for ourselves. I have firsthand experience. I have taken myself from a place of negativity and darkness to a place of possibility. I have watched my newfound passions and work flourish, along with my relationships, personal and otherwise.

This is a different way of looking at things. This just isn't your usual "Be positive" message. This is connecting into the fact that as humans, we have a distinct design in place to help us truly create a good life for ourselves. The foundation of this is to truly feel happy and positive from the inside out, so that what we engage with is affected by our positive energy. Think of the last time you had an encounter with someone who you felt emitted a positive or happy energy? How did it make you feel? How did you react? You truly have the power to combat these negative thought processes (bugs) already in you! Don't you want to be the one truly living in your potential and sharing your positivity with everyone and everything in your life?

THE "AWESOME LIFE" IS WAITING FOR YOU!

Let's get down to business. Thanks for sticking with me. If you have continued reading to this point, then I want to applaud you! It means that you are deeply interested in living your best life.

Side effects of a mind free from negative Thought Bugs may include:
- General feelings of happiness and relaxation
- Genuine connections when meeting people
- A mind free from clutter
- A deep appreciation for the world and people around you
- High levels of productivity
- Willingness to learn new skills
- Gaining more contacts and connections with ease
- Feeling an authentic excitement for projects and self-development
- Being ready to rock your life!

These are just a few of the feelings available to you if you commit to removing negative Thought Bugs from your life, thus strengthening your energy and Aura from the inside out. I wouldn't be here today if I didn't do the work and experience the benefits of being on the other side of the process.

BRING LIGHT TO YOU

My hope for you is to learn how to identify your negative Thought Bugs and stop their process of multiplication. For you to empower yourself with positivity and strengthen your aura. For you to leave feelings of depletion behind and bring your energy back to 100%. For you to share your positive energy with the world and make it a better place!

Never forget: An Awesome Life is within your reach at all times. I believe it. In fact, I will go so far as to say I know it is. I have taken my own life and made it awesome by taking all I have outlined in my work and applying it to myself. Now it is your turn to turn up the positivity in your life and let your Aura shine!

I encourage you to check out my website, www.happinessmountain.com, to receive a free guide on removing your negative energy. In this guide, you will also be given a sneak peek into the app I am developing. The Happiness Mountain™ app will quickly become your new best friend! I developed the Happiness Mountain™ app to be a way to actually track those negative Thought Bugs and coach you to clear your worries and boost your energy levels! By giving you this important tool at your fingertips, I know you will be able to strengthen your energy and basically start living a more happy life! If you haven't guessed already, I love technology and its possibilities for enhancing our lives. I can't wait for you to be one of the first people to try this app and reap its benefits right away at www.happinessmountain.com/app.

BRINGING LIGHT TO YOU SO THAT YOU MAY BRING LIGHT TO THE WORLD

Now that I have given you some insight on how you can truly change your life by changing your own energy, I want to share the ways that Happiness Mountain™ can help you begin to apply these concepts. The process of understanding, application, and execution is key when committing to changing the way your mind functions and, over time, changing your aura.

Now that you know you have the power to change your life via your thoughts, I wonder why you wouldn't want to act now to change your life. Your own personal idea of an awesome life is within reach! I left behind an old way of living and being in order to start on a new path. I am confident that you have the power to do that for yourself as well. We all just need a little help. To be honest, I wish I had connected with these deeper levels of understanding regarding my thoughts and how they affect my life earlier. However, as we all know, timing is everything, especially when it comes to your advancement on both a personal level and a business one. Take this as a sign that it may be time for you to dive into these deep changes. The techniques, once you really begin to understand them, are quite straightforward. I know that you live a busy life and are striving to do your best. However, it takes commitment to change. Why not start now?

Happiness Mountain™ can offer you many tools to get started and help you dive deeper. The first step is easy! I encourage you to head over to my website www.happinessmountain.com to sign up and stay connected to the developments in my work. You will automatically receive an easy to follow guide on how to remove your negative energy, which will be delivered right to your inbox! You will also be given an automatic sneak peek into my app.

THE HAPPINESS MOUNTAIN™ APP

I am constantly inspired by how we connect online through different platforms and technologies. I believe that this can be the start to a great change in how we grow and develop. I designed the app as a convenient way for you to connect to your energy boosting practices on the go. We all spend some time on our phones scrolling and engaging on different platforms. Why not invest that time mindfully instead of mindlessly? The Happiness Mountain™ app, www.happinessmountain.com/app, helps you do that by having the tools you can utilize to boost your own positive energy available at any time!

Features include the following:

- Troubleshooting what is worrying you and replacing that worry with positivity

- Ways to resolve disputes without creating negative energy and affecting your Aura

- Aura boosting activities you can do on daily basis, while tracking your progress with your own private point system

- An emergency toolkit for handling sudden negative situations

- An easy guide to all the Thought Bugs and how to handle them available at a touch of your screen, so that you may continue to learn how you can change your thoughts to more positive ones and keep your positive energy high!

HAPPINESS MOUNTAIN™ FOR KIDS

Calling all parents and anyone who takes care of children! This work isn't just applicable to more mature minds and bodies. It can start when we are young! I am in the process of finishing development on a series of books for children that will cover all the core concepts of my work and Happiness Mountain™, so that we may share these valuable tools and concepts even with the developing minds of the next generation. Of course, there will be interactive games for children as well, because as we all know that some of the best learning happens when we are having fun! This goes for adults too, don't you think? Stay in the loop by connecting with me at www.happinessmountain.com.

MY NEXT BOOK

I am ready to dive deeper and share with you even more in my new book, *Happiness Mountain™: Double Your Happiness, Awesomeness and Spirituality*. In the book we are going to explore deeper than ever before. *Happiness Mountain™* will go more in depth on how you can harness the three levels of energy (Positive/Negative, Aura and Universal) to change your perspective and unlock your perfect life. I want to share with you the techniques and deep processes that will affect all aspects of your life. Remember those 'Negative Thought Bugs' I was talking about earlier? In my new book I will teach you not only how to eliminate them, I want to teach you how to protect yourself from future encounters with 'Negative Thought Bugs' therefore truly creating change in your life for the better. You will also learn techniques on how to recharge your energy, boost your aura and use your new skills for resolving conflicts and affecting your business.

I want you to harness the power of your personal Positive & Aura energies, learn to dance with the Universal energy that is always at your disposable and be able to live at a level of existence that falls in line with your ideal, perfect life. Take a look at the *Happiness Mountain™* diagram on the next page. You can define your perfect life as living with a high level of inner peace, the level of inner happiness. Your Awesome Life and Spiritual Life revolves around being of service to others and helping others. You can live a combination of all levels of the *Happiness Mountain™*. Whatever you personally define as perfection is where you have the power.

```
        /\
       /  \
      /    \
     /      \
    / Spiritual \
   /   Life      \
  /---------------\
 /  Awesome Life   \
/-------------------\
/  Inner Happiness   \
/---------------------\
/ Temporary Fulfillments \
/-------------------------\
/       Rat Race           \
/---------------------------\
```

Happiness Mountain™ created by Amal Indi

Some might argue you cannot have a perfect life. I say you already have a perfect life and it is blocked by negative energy from coming into full fruition. This negative energy can be existing as a low self-esteem bug or a comparison bug. You may define perfect life as comparing to others. You may try to achieve things with craving energy. Please remember: You are already whole, complete and perfect. You cannot access your full power because of the negative energy being generated by your thoughts. When you learn to remove those negative thoughts as I teach you in *Happiness Mountain™*, you will realize how much power you have in life. This will be your turning point to harness the energy to power-up your personal, business and spiritual life! In the book I will give you all the tools and techniques to accomplish that. After reading my new book *Happiness Mountain™* you will be able to shift your life to a new paradigm that is not only accessible but exciting. How do you think it will feel to lead a perfect life? Can you think of even one thing that may change for the better if you decided to investigate how you could crush your negative energies, enhance your positive energies and essentially eliminate future worries from your life? ... Wow! I am excited for you just thinking about it myself! I know the profound changes it created for me in my life and I look forward to hearing how it affects yours.

YOU CAN LEAD AN AWESOME LIFE

My hope for you is to learn how to identify your negative Thought Bugs and stop their process of multiplication. For you to empower yourself with positivity and strengthen your aura. For you to leave feelings of depletion behind and bring your energy back to 100%. For you to share your positive energy with the world and make it a better place!

Never forget: The Awesome Life is within your reach at all times. I believe it. In fact, I will go as so far to say I know it is. I have taken my own life and made it perfect in my eyes by taking all I have outlined in my work and applying it to myself. Again, your negative thoughts may say your life is not perfect, which might include your low self-esteem, cravings, or comparison bugs blocking you. Don't let these bugs create negative energy. Instead, clear them and power-up the personal, business, or spiritual aspects of your life. Never forget you have the power over your own mind- NOT your negative Thought Bugs. Now it is time to power-up the positivity in your life and let your Aura shine!

I encourage you to check out my website, www.happinessmountain.com, for the opportunity to stay connected to the global community of people who have already begun to use this work to boost their positivity and create their

Awesome Life in their personal, business, and spiritual domains. I can't wait for you to begin using The Happiness Mountain™ App to start training your energy to stay positive and even get stronger. Of course, I encourage you to visit www.happinessmountain.com to stay connected and be in the know as to what is coming down the pipeline with this life changing work.

I have dedicated my life to bringing these concepts and work to you. I know you can change your energy and begin to not only affect your own life, but the entire world. I believe deeply that when as many people as possible align their energy to a higher, more positive state, then we can truly make a collective difference. Let's start today!

Amal Indi lives in Vancouver, Canada, and is the founder and CEO of Happiness Mountain™ Inc. After 20 years of working in technology and corporate banking, Amal is on a mission to give people the possibility to live with their full potential in their personal, business, and spiritual domains. He has found innovative techniques and tools to remove negative energy and power up your personal life, business life, and spiritual life. Ultimately, you can make the world a more awesome place for everyone. He believes that technology has the potential to transform the minds and energy of people and facilitate change. Amal wants to help people around the globe live a positive and enriching life through the energy-based tools and techniques of this innovative system he has developed to strengthen your energy and help you live a life full of happiness and potential. Find his story and work at www.happinessmountain.com.

Nobody Got Time For That!

The Ultimate Guide For Smart Money Management

URSULA GARRETT

S ave, save, save! That's all you hear from family, friends and the media. You are strongly encouraged to save, but how are you supposed to save with a low-paying job, high student loan debt, and the rising cost of housing? Something has got to give – and it's usually not you giving to your savings account. Who has time to be broke when you are young and just want to have fun and enjoy your life? I'll tell you who – nobody. Nobody has got time for that, especially you!

Finances absolutely play a huge part in your life choices and opportunities. Money issues consume chunks of your brain power every day. Think of how many times money (or a lack of it) factors into your decisions throughout your fast-paced day. For instance, you schedule a date on Tinder, buy movie tickets on Fandango and make dinner reservation using Open Table, and you haven't even gotten out of bed yet to start your day. You can do this if you have money in your bank account or power (available credit) on your credit card. Yes, either method of payment will get you what you want right now – one is a smart choice and the other, not so much. You must make smart choices regularly, there is no getting around it.

Size does matter, especially when it refers to your bank account. I want you to recognize that money underwrites the type of life you live and the lack of it means you're not living the life you want to be living. You are forced to make hard choices about what you can afford or what you have to give up. Having limited options make you feel as if your life is less than it could be. Smart money management is the key to your financial goals and personal goals aligning.

Once you recognize that the choices you make with your finances are either limiting your options or providing you opportunities, you can start being more proactive with your finances. First, it is important for you to understand how easy it is to handle your personal business, so you can create real changes that will significantly impact your life.

Two of my five daughters are about the same age, 26 (not twins just a blended family). Throughout their lives, they have taken different paths and made different choices. They are in their mid-twenties now and both spend more than they should, however, one is contributing to a retirement plan and has money go directly from her paycheck into a savings account. The other one lives paycheck to paycheck, has no retirement savings, no personal savings, and is regularly subsidized by her parents. Three guesses which one has more opportunities to live the life she wants, and the first two guesses don't count. While they each had similar opportunities, their individual choices have dictated their current circumstances.

"I am not a product of my circumstances. I am a product of my decisions."

- Stephen Covey

It's a bit of a mystery why you make some of the decisions you make and that's especially true when it comes to your finances. I can tell you from experience that a crystal ball, mesmerizing though it may be, is not where you will find those answers. How often have you made poor financial choices in the moment, only to later regret them and wonder how you got into this situation again? Well, I'm here to tell you that it doesn't matter how or why, what matters is what you do to fix it and make sure it never happens again.

If you have ever paid attention to political elections, then you know how easily you can be fooled by your assumptions, fears and false intuitions. I say this to help you understand that listening to others' opinions about what you should do won't help you reach your goals. Making a plan and following through will.

Which is why I find it useful to understand some principle concepts when you make decisions about money. This is besides, of course, the regular practices of following a budget, saving, investing and avoiding most kinds of debt, factors that I will discuss as part of the steps for smart money management.

These four concepts are the foundation you need for your decision-making process when you are creating your budget or making the decisions about those investments and savings plans. They need to factor into all your financial decisions, because they will help keep you from sabotaging your financial stability.

1) OPPORTUNITY COSTS

No matter what you do or the opportunities that you pursue, there is always going to be a cost. You have to give something to get something. Nothing in life is free. Individually, we get to decide what we are willing to give in exchange. In some circumstances, the price is simply too high, or the payoff is too low to make the deal or take the chance. That threshold is different for everyone and is based on your values.

For example, deciding whether or not to pursue higher education is a decision you make based on your priorities, which could include your financials, your time, and your perception of the value of higher education. Pursuing an advanced degree may take years -- are you willing to put in that amount of time? It could involve giving up other opportunities to finish your degree, but at the same time, the network you build could allow you access to individuals who can create even greater career opportunities in the future. Many individuals choose their university based on the alumni and the type of network they can access for mentors.

Additionally, there is the debt that often comes with pursuing higher education. Are you willing to put yourself into that kind of debt, the type of debt that will take years to pay off? Many individuals see their degree as a doorway to career advancement in a specific field or as a way to pursue the type of work that they are passionate about. For them, the cost of the degree in terms of finances and time is worth it, because they see that degree as an investment in their long-term financial future.

Those two daughters I mentioned earlier, one went to college and has a degree in business and some student loan debt. The other worked part-time jobs and traveled to visit friends she met on the internet. One daughter wanted a college degree and was willing to sacrifice four years of her life, accumulate debt (she considered it as an investment) and forego immediate travel opportunities. The other daughter thought that price was too high. This isn't a matter of right or wrong but a matter of what you are willing to give to get what you want. Here is a general rule of thumb: The bigger the opportunity, the greater the cost or sacrifice to achieve it.

Every decision that you make has all those considerations and it is up to you to give them all a voice before you make your decision. At the same time, your priorities need to guide those smaller financial decisions that we all make throughout the day. Many of your long-term goals are going to be impacted by your short-term decisions. Therefore, giving yourself guidelines for daily spending based on your priorities will help you to reach those goals. Still, not everything can be quantified in terms of your return on investment, as I will explore next.

2) SUNK COSTS

What is sunk cost? This is money you can't get back -- a non-refundable airline ticket, for example. There are certain expenses that you will have throughout your life that are not going to bring a tangible return on investment. In fact, they are likely going to result in nothing more than an enjoyable experience or a pleasant memory. It can be easy to get into a mindset that has you spending far beyond what you may have budgeted or prioritized because you value the experience, but it can put you in a financial bind later. The idea here is that you need to keep sunk costs in proper perspective. It's easy to start thinking, "Well, I've already spent $100, so what's another $25?" My mother always told me not to throw good money after bad. She taught me to understand the concept of sunk costs long before I took a business class. You have got to be willing to walk away sometimes and keep the money in your pocket for other investment opportunities.

Once something is paid for, and cannot be refunded, it shouldn't impact your future financial decisions. It is a "sunk" cost, i.e. water under the bridge, and no matter what you do in the future you won't ever get it back. Therefore, you can't allow yourself to get hung up on the moments where you spent money in a way that didn't fall into your overall financial plan. In the end, you have to accept that sunk costs are going to happen and make your peace with them. Recognize that you will buy emotionally and defend rationally, even if that might not always be wise. There are costs that are simply not recoupable.

Regrets over sunk costs can make it harder to move forward, leaving you vulnerable to make other choices that you may not have otherwise made. Do not allow yourself to fall into the downward spiral. Negative thoughts often breed more negative thoughts, especially if you continue to dwell on them. The same can be said for financial decisions. When you focus on your bad financial decisions, you may find yourself repeating them, because that is your focus.

It is important to keep yourself focused on ways to improve your financial decisions and keep them in line with your financial plan. Yes, you might regret a decision, but make the conscious choice not to dwell on it. Instead, learn from it and move forward. Life, especially when it comes to finances, is a series of learning experiences. The better you are at accepting the lessons, the better decisions you will be able to make in the future. I find inspiration and humor in the lyrics of one of my favorite songs by Chumbawamba, "I get knocked down, but I get up again, you're never gonna keep me down."

Now that you have that mindset (and that song stuck in your head), you can keep yourself from making financial decisions based on your sunk costs and focus on maximizing your earnings. That starts by focusing on finding the right investments for you. With that in mind, let's talk about the Rule of 72.

3) QUICK INTEREST CALCULATIONS USING THE RULE OF 72

One of your biggest concerns about an investment should be, "What am I going to get out of this?" While you wouldn't want to ask that of a date, it's perfectly acceptable, in fact it's expected, to ask that of a potential investment. All of us want a way to determine the upside of a financial opportunity. Now there are several ways to analyze a financial investment, but it often comes down to how long it will take for an investment to pay off. Want to double your holdings? The Rule of 72 can tell you how long it will take, based on the specific interest rate. Just divide 72 by the interest rate to learn how long it will take to double your initial investment.

For example, if you are looking at an investment with an interest rate of 6 percent, then 72 divided by 6 gets you 12 years. You can then take that information and use it to determine if that timeframe will work with your overall financial plan. Granted, you may find that other factors will play a part in determining your return as well, but it is important to have an idea of what you can expect before you put money into an investment.

This is a rough estimate, of course, but it's pretty effective. Recognize that you might find that a return is going to take significantly longer to make you money. So even if you find it an interesting opportunity, you may opt to not invest in order to take advantage of a different opportunity that will give you a faster return on your money.

In fact, you can also turn the equation around to determine the interest rate you are looking at if someone promises to double your returns in a set amount of time. Twice as much money in 12 years? Divide 72 by 12 and you get an interest rate of 6 percent. This rule lets you evaluate investment opportunities quickly and decide where to put your money in a way that will help you to grow your investments to meet long-term financial goals.

Keep in mind, future earnings are not something that you can count on, so how you use the dollars that you have now are going to have greater weight than potential earnings. You know that old saying, "Don't count your chickens before the eggs hatch."

4) THE TIME VALUE OF MONEY

According to this concept, a dollar you receive today is worth more than a dollar you will get tomorrow. You will have opportunity to invest that dollar immediately and begin earning more revenue from it (and also avoid losing value because of inflation).

It is important to recognize that money from your investments needs to be put to work. Don't be quick to spend it. Making frivolous or useless purchases means you are making a choice to spend on meaningless things and activities and in doing so, you are draining your ability to invest and grow. Focus on how you can essentially create a chain of investments, all working to grow an income stream for you to use in retirement or even for a big purchase that is part of your financial plan (think a house or car). Growth is a long-term process and it is imperative that you do make the time for it.

When you are waiting for an investment to pay off, then you are waiting for your money to work for you. One of the ways that you can save money is by limiting your interest payments. When you are making money from investments, which is then reinvested, you create an income stream that can allow you to pay cash for items, or put down a larger down payment, thus helping to reduce those interest payments, or eliminate them altogether.

Again, this helps you make certain calls about your purchases -- and your income. It's the old "one bird in the hand is worth two in a bush" theory in action for your wallet.

These four concepts have served me well over the years. Now let's focus in on the five steps that will help you to remain financially sound as you invest and grow your income to meet your financial goals.

WHY MONEY MATTERS

Before I talk about the steps, I want you to understand that money has a place and purpose in your life. Whatever adventures or experiences you want to have, you are going to need money to do it. That money is also going to be a key part of fulfilling your life's purpose, simply because money is a resource that can help you get things done. Regardless of if your goal in life is to have a non-profit that helps others or to create a company to bring a product or process to market, the truth is that money will be a resource that you need.

Since you and I can agree on that, let's start talking about your financial goals by first talking about your life goals.

STEP 1 - BUDGETING: YOUR PERSONAL BUSINESS PLAN

You have goals you want to accomplish, experience, and create in this life. This is simply a reality we all share. By defining your goals, you are able to determine what financial moves are necessary to achieve them. Too often, personal goals are overlooked or under-appreciated when creating a financial plan. Your personal goals and your financial plan need to be in sync for you to be successful at achieving either one.

For instance, if you know that your financial plan is going to allow you to achieve your personal goals, then it will help you maintain the excitement and vision you have for your life. This knowledge will help keep up the momentum during tough times or difficult circumstances when you are making sacrifices.

Budgeting should be the first part of your financial plan, because it will show the money you have coming in and going out. Once you understand your cash flow, then you have all the information you need to make a sound financial plan. Your budget will allow you to make good choices about how you want to use your money and where you can make changes in your spending habits to align your personal goals with your financial goals.

As part of that budgeting process, you need to look at the choices you make on a daily basis. Consider that if you take out that Tinder date on Saturday night maybe you can't afford to play golf on Sunday. If you really want to golf, then maybe you have to Netflix and chill with $1 bottles of beer or a $7 bottle of wine and takeout pizza instead of your dinner and a movie date. We all have to make choices. Just make sure your choices are good choices. You may find that you are sabotaging yourself by the financial decisions you make every day.

The good news is that you don't have to try to figure out a budget on your own or hire a professional to do it for you. All you need is that device that sometimes acts as another appendage – your cell phone. Yes, there is another reason that your cell phone is your best friend because there's an app for that (for budgeting, that is). Actually, there are several apps for that, you just have to choose the one that works best for you.

I use Mint to track my personal bank accounts, credit cards, investments and bills – it creates a budget based on my income and expenses and reminds me when I have a payment due date. I love that my whole financial life is accessible in one place and that I can monitor activity at a glance. One of my daughters uses Clarity Money, which has similar features plus the added benefit of helping to cancel unwanted subscriptions. With an app, you won't have to wonder if you are spending too much money shopping or eating out, you can see it in full color. Knowledge is power, and this knowledge can be used to change your spending behavior to match your financial goals.

For instance, think about that $5 cup of coffee you stop to buy every morning to start your day. That money falls into the sunk costs pot, because you are not getting that money back and it is not working for you. Imagine how much money you could save if you took that $5 per day for a year and saved or invested it – you would have more than $1,825. Going back to those two daughters of mine, one likes to buy and play internet games, a lot – can you guess which one? I'll tell you it's not the one that uses Clarity Money. If you are having trouble saving to meet your long-term goals, then it might be worth exploring using an app to help you get control of your spending.

It is not about giving up your lifestyle, but making your lifestyle adhere to your financial priorities, instead of letting your lifestyle dictate your priorities. Everyone has time to know their money.

Part of achieving any financial goal is to create a nest egg of funds to work with, which serves as a basis for your investment portfolio. Using your budget, you can designate a specific percentage to go into your savings.

STEP 2 – SAVING

The point of saving is to create a financial resource that you can use to build your income streams. These income streams can be diversified, but the point is that saving has to be a priority in order to improve your financial situation and allow you to reach your goals. Here are just a few reasons why saving is important.

1. You have a nest egg for emergencies. Time and time again, financial emergencies have sunk individuals who appear to be doing well, simply because they had nothing to fall back on. Once it happens, they have a financial issue, one that can have a ripple effect across other areas of their lives. Point blank, having an emergency, such as an unexpected car repair or house repair, should not financially sink you. Experts recommend that your savings for emergency needs to cover six months of your living expenses. Once you reach that goal, keep saving a set amount to grow your emergency fund. If you have to use some of it for an emergency, then replace it as soon as possible.

2. You can save for larger purchases. You know that paying cash for items can save you money in the long run, because you won't pay interest on top of the purchase cost. When you designate savings for specific

purchases, it allows you to reach your financial goals without acquiring payments. Plus, once you make that big purchase, you can start saving for the next big item or event.

3. You can save to invest to build income streams. Once you have achieved your emergency savings goal, start building a savings that is specifically for investments. These funds should not be used for any other purpose, allowing you to adjust the rate of return to meet your goals.

Clearly, saving is important because it gives you a stepping stone to meet your financial needs and personal dreams. Now, I want to transition to the exploring the possibilities that you can create with a savings that was started for investing.

STEP 3 – INVESTING

When you reach the point that you have started an investment savings account, you have plenty of opportunities. From stocks and bonds to direct investing in a business, you have multiple ways to grow your investment dollars. That being said, it is important to choose investments that fall in line with your goals and your risk tolerance level.

For instance, if you are at the beginning of your career, you might find yourself more inclined to look for high return, risky investments. Why? Many of those who are younger see time on their side and recognize that they have time to recover from a loss. Alternately, as you reach specific benchmarks or get closer to achieving your financial goals, you will start to make less risky investments.

Another potential scenario is that you are planning to get married or start a family, in which case, you might be more concerned with the risk of losing the primary financial provider. In a case like this, you may be more interested in investing in a disability or life insurance policy or even starting a college fund. After all, not all investments are created equal.

Where you are in your life can play a large part in what type of investments you choose to take on. Additionally, you might take on investments that are less time-consuming because they give you the ability to do more of what you enjoy. On the other hand, you might want to be more hands-on in your investments, so that may be a factor in the types of investments you choose.

Your investment plan should be personalized to you and designed to meet your needs. I want you to recognize that working with a financial advisor can help you to determine the best investments for you.

Many of the individuals I work with even consider investing in themselves, which means starting their own business. If you want to explore your entrepreneurial spirit, that can be a great way to invest and see your returns grow, using your investment dollars and sweat equity. Again, I encourage you to put any investment up against your financial plan. Ask yourself the hard questions about whether it will work towards accomplishing your goals. Doing so is critical to keeping you focused and on the path to achieving both your financial and personal goals. Just keep in mind that it takes time to grow and any time frames set by you can be changed, especially if the situation changes.

STEP 4 – AVOIDING MOST KINDS OF DEBT

Debt can drown you financially and make it difficult for you to achieve your financial goals. When you look at your budget, do you see areas where you are spending money on payments regularly? That is money which is not being used to create income streams or to reach your financial goals.

Be picky when you are choosing to take on debt. I recommend that you only finance things that will bring in money or pay for themselves. It's okay to finance your education because you expect your education to yield you a higher paying career. Do not finance your vacation because you will have nothing but memories to show for it. You can pay for your business advertising with a credit card but not your groceries. Avoid running up your credit cards, leaving yourself strapped with payments. The interest payments can quickly exceed your budget and be a drain. Use the cash in your bank account to pay for your living expenses because the interest on credit cards is usually greater than the interest you earn on money deposited in the bank.

Some debt can be beneficial and preferable because it shares the risk. I am talking about debt that involves investing. For instance, if you are building a real estate portfolio of rentals and you have $100,000 to invest, you might find that you choose to split that $100,000 into down payments for five properties instead of just buying one for $100,000. The reason is that you can increase your cash flow across five properties and they can also cover their own overhead. In the meantime, you are creating equity that you can tap into later to purchase more properties. The point is that you want to use your investment cash to maximize your income opportunities. Do not limit yourself because you want to avoid all debt – some debt can be good.

When weighing your debt options, be sure to look at interest rates. Do not feel as if you are limited to one lender or one financing option. Shop around and make sure that you get the lowest possible rate for your debt with the best payment plan to meet your investment needs. Also, make sure that any investment purchased with debt is going to have a positive cash flow. Some investments may not have a positive cash flow initially but will overtime as the debt is paid down. For other investments, it is the value which grows over time that offsets the lack of a positive cash flow.

Again, it is important to work with a professional who can help you determine what types of debt you want to take on regarding your investments and what debt you want to avoid.

In the end, this step is mostly focused on helping you to avoid debt that drains you financially, without giving you any type of return. Think about the cost of those daily coffees. The focus of this step needs to be on defining the lifestyle you want and then investing in order to be able to afford it. If you opt to live a lifestyle that drains your investments, you could be shortchanging yourself for the future, thus limiting your ability to reach your dreams.

STEP 5 – EVALUATE AND ASSESS: ONGOING PROCESS

I call this step, "the shit happens" part of your plan. Yes, it would be nice if life happened exactly as we planned it, but real life is no fairy tale. The reality is that you made a plan based on the life you wanted to live and all the messy stuff that got in your way is why you had contingency plans, emergency funds and cushions built into your plan. Shit happens, and you deal. You deal by adapting to your new situation. Update your plan as if it is a living, breathing organism.

For instance, you had an accident that kept you from working for six months. That would be both physically and financially draining. This is only a temporary setback. Now you need to reset your goals to achieve your plans, because you may need to focus on rebuilding instead of growth. Still, the point is to make adjustments that help you achieve your goals, thus not allowing the circumstances to overwhelm you and derail your finances permanently.

This need to make adjustments also applies to your investments. I recommend at least once per quarter that you review your investments to make sure they are performing as expected. You don't want to waste your resources on underperforming investments.

Are there areas you might want to expand even further, or do you need to eliminate some investments because they no longer fit your financial goals? Doing these reviews regularly can help you to keep your financial life on track with your personal life. When the two are in sync, then you will find that your life continues to improve. This harmony makes it possible to achieve what you want, no matter the setbacks you might occasionally encounter.

Keep in mind that evaluating and assessing will always be ongoing processes. The fluidity of life is that you can create plans, but events may alter those plans or even offer you new opportunities and experiences that you might not have even considered.

It is important to keep your mind open, both to new investments and to new experiences and opportunities in your personal life. They often can dovetail together more than you ever realize.

Financially, your world is built on the decisions that you make throughout your life. Always know the direction you want to go before you start your journey. When you make decisions without direction, your life will be like a boat without a rudder. It goes all over but doesn't actually get anywhere. The waves take the boat in multiple directions without a clear destination.

I want you to define your path and then work in harmony with that by making choices to complement it. Even with a defined path, it can be easy to make decisions that run contrary to your goals, as I discussed earlier in this chapter. When I work with individuals, I help them to not only define their path, but also to determine the types of goals that align with their paths. Then, I can help them to find the right investments and set financial goals to help them go further on that path.

Growth happens by learning from those people who inspire you to do and be more. We all have time to learn and grow.

Please email Ursula Garrett at ugarrett@cpagarrett.com or visit her website www.cpagarrett.com

Simple Steps for Big Results in Boosting Heart Health

RALSTON POWELL

"First say to yourself what you would be: and then do what you have to do."
— Epictetus

It strikes like lightning, and it steals loved ones from their families. It is the number one killer of men and women in Western societies; twelve million people die from it each year around the world. While some of its warning signs are obvious, it can come disguised as flu, headache, or just plain fatigue.

Some people have no symptoms and do not see it coming. They are oblivious to the damage that is already done until they are at severe risk of a catastrophe. It can happen at any time, even when they are at rest. If you do not act fast enough or seek help within minutes, it can be fatal.

What am I talking about here? What is this disease that takes lives by stealth, which can recur even when you've recovered from it?

A heart attack.

How many of you have lost a loved one, a friend, or a colleague to a heart attack? Sadly enough, there are many of us in these ranks. It is clear that people are getting sick and dying even at a young age. In fact, I first became concerned about the rising incidence of both heart disease and cancer when a member of my church died of Leukemia. This man was young, approximately 30 years old with a wife and young children. At the time, anyone who was diagnosed with cancer of the blood felt a sense of hopelessness. The second time I felt a sense of concern was when I heard of the death of a young man at a prominent company that I would visit daily. His diagnosis was a massive heart attack. Following that, a friend and co-worker who was having problems with his heart went on vacation to Guyana; in the heat, he suffered a massive heart attack and died. These experiences made me concerned enough to do research, and I found out that heart disease is stated to be North America's number one killer. People from all walks of life can be affected.

Heart disease is commonly reported among those who are physically unfit, carry too much weight, who smoke and drink heavily, and who are eating fat-rich foods. Yet it is no longer just the plight of middle-aged men. Women are just as susceptible, especially after menopause.

Tragically, there are now stories that heart disease is striking the seemingly healthy. You can be a marathon runner, observe a low-calorie diet, have manageable cholesterol, and you can still suffer a catastrophic heart attack without any notice or warning signs.

WHAT IS A HEART ATTACK?

Your heart is no bigger than a fist, but it is your strongest organ, and it works tirelessly from the time you take your first breath to your last. It is made of cardiac muscle, a specialized muscle that only exists in the heart, and, unlike muscles in our legs or arms, the cardiac muscle never tires.

The heart works to pump life-giving oxygen and nutrients in the blood to every part of your body. On average, it beats between 60-100 times per minute at rest. When you work out or are feeling anxious or angry, your heart beats more quickly.

Feeding the heart with blood are the coronary arteries. When there is too much cholesterol in the bloodstream, it gets deposited on the inner linings of these blood vessels, just like rust on the insides of old plumbing. These deposits, called plaque, build up and block oxygen from getting to the heart.

Decreased blood flow causes chest pain, angina, or shortness of breath. A complete blockage of blood flow can damage or destroy part of the heart muscle. Typical symptoms of an attack are anxiety, sweating, chest pain, stiffness or discomfort in the upper body, nausea, and stomach pain.

A person can survive a heart attack due, in part, to significant improvements in medical treatment, yet the statistics are ugly. More than 60% of people who suffer a heart attack die before getting the medical help that they need.

WHAT'S THE GOOD NEWS HERE?

The good news is that a heart attack is absolutely preventable. And its damage is reversible. If you've suffered the disease before, you can empower yourself to make sure you'll never be victim to another attack again. You can do so with minimal or zero drug use or surgical interventions, such as a coronary bypass or having stents placed in your arteries to improve blood flow.

You can lead a healthier life by making easy lifestyle changes. These adjustments are so simple you can see results within a month. Not only that, but you also reduce the risks against you by more than half.

Pretty good news, isn't it?

Changing the way you live is far more effective in prevention and repair than any number of drugs or tubes put into your body. Treating only the symptoms or the risks is taking the short-view, and that is why, once your doctor prescribes medication, you are on it for the rest of your life. You can stop playing the victim and take back control of your own life. By investing some time and committing to making the changes, you can protect yourself from this devastating disease and live life fully.

HEALTH IS OUR BIRTHRIGHT

It is time for a paradigm shift in the way we look at the prevention of heart disease and its therapy for rehabilitation. We must go beyond the conventional attitudes and treatments that limit how we can live healthier lives.

The first step we must take is to change the way we look at our health. I've always firmly believed that health is our birthright. Our bodies are wonderful, complex, finely-tuned instruments. There're no two ways of saying it - it is a miracle!

Picture this. You make a small cut on your finger when you're cutting vegetables. You may run tap water over the finger to stop the bleeding, pour hydrogen peroxide on it, and apply a band-aid. Since it was a small and superficial cut, you're completely healed within a few days. Voila!

But what has taken place without conscious intervention from you is a sequence of healing events. The moment the skin is cut, the blood vessels feeding blood to the area miraculously reduce blood flow to the injured area, like turning off the tap. Next, platelets rush to the scene. They have been alerted to the emergency by enzymes released from the damaged blood vessels. The platelets clot together to form a plug that becomes a scab to stop the blood vessel from bleeding further. In the meantime, signals are sent out to more platelets to come help at the site of the damage.

When the bleeding is under control, the constricted blood vessels open up again, this time bringing important white blood cells to destroy any germs or infections that may have gotten into the body through the wound. Then the body concentrates on healing and rebuilding. The skin on both sides of the cut stretches to meet in the middle, forming a scar, which may or may not disappear as the body adds more collagen to the area. The finger is almost as good as new.

Notice that I said all of this happened without any conscious thought on your part. That's because you are gifted with a terrific immune system with enormous healing power, which orchestrates events to repair and renew your body even as you're reading this sentence.

TIME TO GET SMART ABOUT HEART HEALTH

Why does disease happen then? When we are out of balance, both physically and emotionally, we suppress our immune functions. We turn our body from its natural alkaline state in which disease cannot flourish to an acidic state, which is ripe ground for illnesses like heart diseases and diabetes.

We need to look at health as being much more than just being free of disease. We should look at health as the perfect mind-body balance and the platform from which we can reach our highest potential, our greatest creativity, and lasting happiness.

At this point, I wish to reiterate that power lies within you.

What if there is a history of heart disease in your family? Doesn't it run in the genes? It is mistaken thinking to blame it on a shared heritage. Heart attacks are caused by how the environment affects your genes. So, really, it is what you eat, how much or little you exercise, how you handle stress, and environmental toxins that cause hypertension, high cholesterol, and other imbalances such as high blood sugar that increase the risk of a heart attack.

By turning from victim to someone who takes control with courage and determination, you will make healthy choices, add beneficial foods, exercises, therapies, and natural supplements to your lifestyle. Remember to be kind to yourself and take baby steps, but also congratulate yourself for every accomplishment, no matter how small.

CUT BACK RISK FACTORS

The number of things that make us more vulnerable to heart attacks are called risk factors. Research shows that poor lifestyle choices heighten some of these risk factors, including:

o   Smoking
o   Unhealthy diet

o   Insufficient exercise

o   Chronic stress

These unfortunate lifestyle decisions lead to physical problems such as high blood pressure, high blood sugar, and a high level of blood fats. High blood pressure forces the heart to work harder than it should, causing it to weaken faster over time. High blood sugar speeds up the narrowing and the hardening of the arteries. We have already discussed the damage to the heart from high cholesterol levels.

Unrelieved stress from feeling anxious, lonely, isolated, or angry also causes significant damage. It is hard to accept that stress can be the single trigger for a heart attack. But stress creates that string of events that can lead to that one, catastrophic heart attack. Stress raises cholesterol levels, aggravates blood sugar imbalances, and elevates blood pressure, all of which make the blood more likely to clot.

In plain speak, the more risk factors there are in your life, the higher the risk you run of a heart attack.

SIMPLE STEPS, BIG RESULTS

There are steps you can take, starting now. It is better for you to add one simple change every day rather than attempt to do everything at once and give up down the road because you're overwhelmed by having to do too much at any one time.

Here are a few suggestions of what you can do:

1. Stop smoking. You reduce the odds of a heart attack from the very moment you stop using tobacco.

2. Move it, move it, move it. Medical literature recommends exercising 30 minutes or more several days of the week. But in a pinch, even ten minutes of intense physical exercise goes a long way to making a difference. Take the stairs rather than the escalator, take a walk during lunch, get off at an earlier stop and walk the last few blocks to work or home.

3. Eat heart-healthy foods. Five servings of fruit and vegetables are a daily must, and if you must snack, pick vegetables like carrots, cucumbers, peppers, or fruit. Avoid the temptation to indulge in a sugar-rich pastry. Other heart-healthy foods are lean meats, fish, low-fat dairy, and beans.

4. Load up on antioxidants. These are the nutrients that repair daily damage to your arteries. Fruits and vegetables contain antioxidants. Green tea is another source of antioxidants; it has several powerful antioxidants that reduce cholesterol levels.

5. Cut back on fats. Reduce trans fats from margarine and avoid saturated fats, which are fats that turn solid at room temperature such as butter, cheese, and animal fats. Use olive oil as a substitute for butter or margarine and make sure you buy cold-pressed extra virgin oil as it has more of the healthy antioxidants.

6. Support with supplements. Pick antioxidant vitamin supplements such as Vitamin E and B vitamins, including B6 and folic acid. Add healthy omega-3 fats to your diet by sprinkling a couple of tablespoons of pre-ground flaxseed to your salad, smoothies, or cereal. Flaxseed oil, like fish oil, has been shown in studies to reduce certain cardiac risk factors.

7. Get regular check-ups. Consult with your doctor, but also broaden your choices by seeking advice from natural therapy providers such as a naturopath or nutritionist. No one knows it all, and you must take

responsibility for your own health. Conduct research and catch up on the latest reading.

8. Get good quality sleep. When we sleep, we give the body time and space to carry out the repair work to heal and to boost good health. Insufficient sleep is linked to weight gain, high blood pressure, and other heart disease risk factors. Sufficient sleep is defined as between seven to nine hours.

BOOST HEALING BY CREATING A HEALING ENVIRONMENT

Reducing stress is a major ingredient in the recipe for good health, so find ways to relieve stress in your life. Rethink a tendency to overwork in the office and sort out your priorities so you do not get too upset when work is frustrating. Build support groups and nurture strong relationships. Emotional support from friends and family are stress buffers.

Stack up on stress management tools. There are so many relaxation techniques available to any of us, such as yoga, Tai Chi, Qigong, acupuncture, or guided meditations. Yoga has become commonplace with many community centers offering classes. Acupuncture is recommended as a natural remedy to rebalance the body's energy flow, improve circulation, and blood flow to the heart.

Meditation has been shown to lower cholesterol and reverse any thickening of the carotid arteries. You can join meditation groups, download soothing music, and even find free guided meditations online which you can follow within the sanctuary of your own home. The idea is to have fun and experiment to see which one resonates best with you. Be committed and consistent with the relaxation techniques of your choice; you are making great strides towards better health.

Here's another tip: Do you know how health and beauty spas get you to slow down and chill out by playing slow, meditative music? Notice that they do not have loud rock-and-roll because meditative melodies slow the heart rate, while loud and fast beats rev up our natural heart rate. Prepare a playlist of soft, soothing music to help you take it down a notch.

PAY HEED TO THE MIND-BODY CONNECTION

Health is not just a state of the body, it is also a state of mind. Our bodies react to what we think and how we feel, and the mind-body connection is constantly in play.

It shouldn't surprise you that one of the best mind-body exercises is to have a good laugh. Laughter is the best medicine. We've all heard this before, and it is such a common saying that we often overlook how true the advice is. When you laugh out loud, you can't stay depressed, angry, or frustrated. In fact, a good belly laugh turns these negative emotions on their head.

When you're laughing until your sides hurt, you're doing many good things for your body: You're giving the T-cells a good boost. These are special white blood cells that are crucial to the immune system. They regulate the immune response or directly swoop down on infected cells. The T-cells need to be activated, and a good laugh will do precisely that.

Laughing promotes a sense of well-being. Endorphins are the feel-good chemicals that are produced from exercise. Laughter produces a healthy dose of endorphins and also contributes to an overall positive outlook on life. Those who have a more positive attitude tend to stay healthier or recover faster.

Your body relaxes for up to 45 minutes after laughing. Furthermore, laughter is contagious. Sharing a laugh with someone lowers barriers, promotes intimacy, and enhances relationships, all of which are good things that boost heart health.

Set your mind towards optimal health and successful healing. The change in attitude may seem like a small step, but before you know it, you've made giant strides towards maintaining a healthy heart.

Break Free From Your Pain Cycle

Winning the Battle and
Conquering Autoimmune Disease

SEEMA GIRI

"It is not a journey of understanding; it is a journey of trust. It is a journey of surrendering every aspect of your soul over to the light."

— Panache Desai

D o you have an autoimmune disease? Did you suffer for years before obtaining a diagnosis? Have you been told there's no cure for your condition? If so, I suggest you look beyond your doctors and dive into the ocean of information that's available today regarding autoimmune conditions. You can also begin your journey back to health, take charge of your recovery by reading this chapter. That's right, I know you can reclaim your life. I've done it, and so can you!

"Sometimes it's controversy; but we all have choices that we make."
— **Solomon Burke**

There's a rising healthcare epidemic today. According to the American Autoimmune Related Diseases Association (AARDA), nearly 50 million Americans have some form of an autoimmune disorder. Business Wire, a Berkshire Hathaway company, has reported, "The global autoimmune diseases treatment market is estimated to grow at a [Compound Annual Growth Rate] CAGR of 3.80 for the forecasted period, and its market value is expected to reach $45.54 billion by 2022, up from $36.41 billion in 2016." Also, the National Institute of Health (NIH) claims that annual direct health care costs for autoimmune diseases are in the range of $100 billion (source: NIH presentation by Dr. Fauci, NIAID). According to the data published by the NIH, autoimmune disorders have been ranked in the top ten types of disorders leading to increasing mortality rates amongst women. These numbers are alarming!

As if this isn't enough, there's evidence today that the government, as well as agriculture and pharmaceutical companies, have been creating controversial dietary guidelines that primarily serve their needs rather than the needs of the people. This has been reported by major news channels, the Huffington Post and Marion Nestle, the consumer activist, nutritionist and academic who specializes in the politics of food and dietary choice. Roberto Ferdman of the Washington Post discusses this concern at length in his exposé "We Don't Know What to Eat." It gets worse. Soda companies are funding 96 health groups in the US—as covered by Time Magazine on Oct. 10, 2016. There's also evidence of an increasing number of illnesses nationally, globally and even in our children today.

So let me ask you, are we really getting objective information for our highest good? I certainly don't think so and it breaks my heart to see how little our lives are valued. What's the difference between lab rats and us? It's not as bad as it could be because there are an equal number of medical doctors, lobbyists, alternative medical practitioners and eastern holistic practitioners doing research and presenting their results. The recent movie "Heal" is a film by Kelly Noonan Gores about the power of the mind to heal the body, featuring Deepak Chopra, Bruce Lipton and Marianne Williamson. The film "Autoimmune Secrets" by Jonathan Otto also comes to mind. Then there's me taking responsibility to share my journey as a member of the global community.

"There are two primary choices in life: to accept conditions as they exist, or accept the responsibility for changing them."
— **Denis Waitley**

The good news is that you and your family don't have to be part of the statistics just mentioned. And you don't have to be affected by propaganda. You simply need to accept responsibility for changing your life and not accept anyone giving you limited information. This is more critical today than ever before.

It's important to make the CHOICE to take control of your health and that of your family. The answer isn't more medication. The answer is becoming more aware and educated. The answer lies in identifying the root cause. I'm passionate about educating you on this topic because life is a collection of precious, irreplaceable moments. Mothers should witness every moment of their children's lives. Children should not be robbed of their childhood. Fathers and husbands should not have to watch their family struggle and feel helpless. Families should not have to go thru the trauma of strained relationships because of lack of trust and differing beliefs. My family and I have lived through this. In Maya Angelou's words, "My mission in life is to not merely survive, but to thrive; and to do so with some passion, some compassion, some humor and some style"

"Our lives begin to end the day we become silent about
things that matter."
— **Martin Luther King Jr.**

Will you join me in creating a revolution to break free from your pain cycle? I hope so. I'm going to share some of my story with you, and then outline the changes you'll need to make on your journey back to health, as well as some resources to help you.

"We are all Working Together; that's the Secret."
— **Sam Walton**

There's a quiet but pervasive problem in the world today. It's a sense of shame resulting from mental and physical health conditions. People feel they can't speak out, that others won't understand—and they're right! This is impacting families; it's impacting men, women and children (who are going to be the leaders of tomorrow). The problem can also be seen as a race to keep up with the acceptable norms of social and economic standards or as we say, "keeping up with the Jones'." Technology has helped increase anxiety with the ease of reach and exposure at the click of a button.

My focus in this chapter is going to be mainly on women in the middle class. Why women? Out of the 50 million Americans that have autoimmune disease 80 percent are women. I believe this is so because we are part of the sandwich generation; we need to take care of elderly parents and children. This leads to compromises in our own health. There just isn't enough time. And, of course, there are the effects of hormonal imbalances. Also, women are the primary caregivers in the family. They're at the centre of the family and have a great influence on everyone else. If we help the women—who are the counselors, the ones who spend the most time with our kids, and to who others constantly come to share their confidences— and they become whole people, what do think will happen to those around them? They're going to change.

Today, the majority of health issues are due to chronic stress, environmental toxicity and chemical toxicity. Our food is genetically modified and our soil is depleted of the essential nutrients. We aren't getting nutrient dense food. And don't forget emotional and mental toxicities. We don't realize the impact of these on our health. My own autoimmune story has primarily arisen from emotional toxicities and food, as you will see as I unfold my experience.

I'll even speak directly to the Indian community. Why? Because as a culture we keep our feelings to ourselves and internalize things quite a bit. The next epidemic is already here and it's psychological in nature. The stress women experience these days is phenomenal. This can be seen throughout society as a whole via school shootings and hate crimes. Resolving these issues requires getting back to basics. We need to slow down, breathe and listen to each other. We need to be authentic, open our hearts and share our issues. The more we reach out to our community, the easier it will be to support each other in coming up with solutions. Once this is done, you can have sustainable energy and health to be able to enjoy what you love to do as a professional or an entrepreneur.

Visit www.seemagiri.com for a free guide on: How to Reduce Stress.

With an autoimmune disease you tend to forget what normal is. There are layers of pain, layers of suppressed and unprocessed emotions—you know, the ones you say are ok but that still bother you in the back of your mind and that limit your life. To reclaim your health, you have to go through these layers, like you would an onion, and you have to reset and recharge at every step. Each layer brings a new insight and wisdom. While you may never return to the "normal" you used to know, you can absolutely create a new normal that is even better than before. This is like keeping your computer running efficiently; you have to begin deleting files that are no longer serving you and clean your hard drive. In the same way, from time to time you need to release your pent up feelings and resentments and allow forgiveness for others and yourself.

"Forgiveness doesn't excuse anyone's actions. Forgiveness stop actions from destroying your heart."
— **Karen Salmansohn**

You need to give yourself permission to let go of hurtful experiences and a painful past. This comes from acknowledging your situation rather than living in denial; taking responsibility and making the change. Master Choa Kok Sui, Founder of Modern Pranic Healing and Arhatic Yoga, states inner forgiveness deals with love and compassion, while outer forgiveness deals with the necessity to create order and justice. While you can forgive internally, the individual still must deal with consequences or punishment. For example, when a child steals for the first time, you can forgive them but still give age appropriate punishment so he or she doesn't steal again. These two types of forgiveness must be balanced, all while coming from a place of love for yourself and the other person. Otherwise the dis-ease manifests into disease.

"The journey of a thousand miles begins with one single step."
— **Lao Tzu**

I lived a life of confinement, isolation and depression for more than 20 years. I was misdiagnosed by multiple doctors for several years with anxiety, depression, stress, chronic fatigue syndrome, psychological issues and was even called a hypochondriac when the test results showed up normal each time. The worst part was that I had started to believe the pain, inflammation and lack of energy were all in my head. Even my family agreed with my doctors, saying that I needed to just get over it; I wasn't the only one in the world who had health issues, and I needed to learn to deal with it better and move on. Eventually, I was on over 26 medications, many of them causing additional side effects. Not a single bottle came with a warning that said, "may cause extreme sexiness" but rather, came with labels that said, "may cause dizziness, heart problems, depression, suicidal thoughts, etc." Many times I felt the side effects were more dangerous than my actual health problems.

The biggest problem with autoimmune disease is that you look perfectly healthy from the outside while you are having a tsunami on the inside that never ends. Life becomes limited to home and doctor visits, but people don't understand why. Secondly, it mimics many diseases that express themselves with lethargy, fatigue, dizziness, sleeplessness and inflammation. Doctors have to rule out numerous options. I was devastated and felt pushed into a corner. I was a burden on my family. The battle had taken so many years I could understand their frustration as caregivers. And even though there was a dim little voice in my head continuously saying there had to be a better way and that I was meant to have a better life, I fell into a deeper depression. I wasn't being heard by anyone and felt the best way to end everyone's misery was to end the problem, me. I had reached my breaking point and attempted suicide. That's how helpless and hopeless I felt. My thinking was that at least then my family could live a life without limits.

Following the suicide attempt, my family started to take me more seriously, particularly my husband, Upendra. I also realized that I did have a larger purpose in life, that I was meant to make a profound contribution to the world. Yet, there was still doubt in my heart. My greatest strengths were perseverance and courage. I had to use these attributes to fight for a life of possibilities and take charge of my recovery. I chose to listen to that tiny voice that said I was meant to have a better life and continued on my quest until I found a young doctor who believed me, took the time to actively listen to me, and finally did some new tests that enabled him to diagnose me with fibromyalgia and rheumatoid arthritis. Hypothyroidism was diagnosed earlier.

My journey to a "new normal" taught me many things. For example, I realized that the doctors were experimenting with different protocols. This knowledge prompted me to do my own experiments, even though my doctors had told me that lifestyle changes wouldn't make any difference to my condition. I had to try. I was encouraged to find that every time I made a decision, the universe always provided the right resources in terms of people and tools.

I first started making changes to my lifestyle with the help of my friend Mrs. Veena Singla, who introduced me to a whole food nutritional supplement, then exercise and personal development. I could tell I was progressing forward, but then I would go two steps backward, sometimes ten. However, I was persistent and consistent in my efforts to get well.

Because I had lost so much precious time, I hired several coaches to achieve my goals faster—the best investment I ever made in myself. Through their tested systems, life experiences and the perfect balance of empathy, ability to show me my blind spots, and not allowing me to hide, I got unbelievable results quickly. As I continued my journey, working with various therapists, counselors and coaches, I realized how many suppressed and unprocessed emotions I had bottled up inside. These were tough and scary to get through. It took several years of processing and removing layer after layer of emotion, but I managed to get closer to the core of the onion. There were some key pivotal moments that really impacted my life, but I kept peeling away those layers, one at a time.

> *"We didn't realize we were making memories, we just knew we were having fun."*
> — **Winnie The Pooh**

My problems began early in life. My parents were strict. They focused on excellence and were always setting new benchmarks (it was more like a sliding benchmark), that made me feel I could never reach their high standards and which led me to believe I wasn't good enough. My parents' constant pressure changed my basic nature, and I became a quiet introvert who kept to myself. You see, I was a naturally outgoing child who was unafraid of strangers (I loved to go on adventures and talk to all the people I would meet). But my behaviour scared my parents. Being in a country where language was a barrier and in a culture we didn't really understand, there were barriers my parents saw that I didn't see. To me, the locals were just people with a different skin color and language. My parents, however, felt I would be safer if I was quiet and controlled. I was disciplined constantly. I used to get a lot of punishments—from scolding to being grounded to taking away my partner in crime, my bike. This is when I discovered the bus. I started taking the bus to different parts of Berlin, the city in Germany where I lived. There would be times I would even come home at 10 or 11 p.m. I know, I know a seven-year-old should not come home so late, but it didn't phase me, as soon as my punishment was up I would do the same thing. I was hungry for adventures and expeditions! I could not stay in the box and have a life with limits.

Even in India, my playmates weren't limited to children but included monkeys, goats and cows. I was born in Shimla, India, a small town located in the middle ranges of the Himalayas. It's the capital city of Himachal Pradesh. Shimla is a lovely hill station that was the summer capital during the British ruling. I spent a considerable amount of time in the village with my grandparents where I had unlimited time to play. I've had a cow ram its horn into my stomach and pin me against the side of the house. I was bitten by a monkey. And I would hang the kids (baby goats) in the branches of our tree and leave them there (don't worry someone would get them down). This used to be all in a day's work. Now that I have children myself, I realize that I was a handful. My children really had a hard time in getting away with many things. My son, Aman, was equally as determined and managed to challenge me.

There are other significant traumas that have impacted my health, some from which I am still healing and find difficult to talk about. These unpleasant experiences led me to believe that due to the color of my skin and being a girl I wasn't good enough and should be invisible. At one point I was beaten so badly that I almost fainted and was covered in blood. I was also accused of stealing a pencil box, where the teacher pinned me against the wall and screamed in my face. These things happened in Owings Mills, MD, where I was the only Indian in the class. Then in Amherst, MA, when

I was ten years old, I endured the most traumatic experience in my life, one that would shape the rest of my future. It left me numb and speechless. I felt that the ground I was standing on was pulled from underneath me. I had nowhere to turn, no one to talk to, no one to believe me. I went thru life like a zombie. I wouldn't even feel the burn of scalding tea on my hand. I believed that I deserved bad things to happen to me.

I became secluded and was a total introvert, limiting my life to only school and home. I internalized a lot of my feelings. My parents couldn't really understand what I was going through. Sometimes I attempted to share my feelings, but I was told I was not supposed to feel that way and to study harder. My parents were working very hard to make a good living and provide a good life for us. They were also supporting my grandparents and my father's younger brother in India. My mother also started working retail on weekends. So that made me the babysitter for my two younger brothers. I didn't want to add to their stress.

About the time we moved to Germany I began the unexplainable manifesting of swollen hands and arms. Then a problem with my hip put me in the hospital for a month. They couldn't explain the issue. Again, we did the medical dance with the doctors: x-rays, tests, etc., with no logical explanations.

At first, I lived a double life. I had to be one way at home in front of my parents and another way at school to try to be accepted. At home I was quiet and invisible. At school I was more extroverted. But, eventually, I succumbed and lost connection to myself. I finally opened the box myself, stepped into it, sat down and closed the flaps. I lived life within the prescribed limit. If I liked the kind of things my father did, then life was easy. If it was anything outside of his wishes, it wasn't allowed. He had a certain idea of how he wanted life, family and kids to be. It was our job to fit in.

Over the years my health continued to be problematic, and I would see a series of doctors. They would do the same tests that would produce normal results. By the time I was in my 20's and married, I was sleeping 16 to 17 hours per day, and when I did get up, I felt like I had been hit by a transport truck. I was going from doctor to doctor to doctor, and it got to the point where I couldn't do the one-hour commute to and from work. I would fall asleep anywhere, even while driving. Now I was really beginning to think that I wasn't human. How can one have so many health issues/incidents without any explanations? I went wild in my imagination with the possibilities. The doctors were able to identify hypothyroidism fairly quickly. When I found out that there really was something tangibly wrong with me, I broke down in the doctor's office and cried. Six months later I was back in the same office because I was still having inflammation and pain. By now I was seeing Dr. Rusk at University of Pennsylvania. He was the first doctor who believed me, and who said my pain was real (that was another hug the doctor, crying moment) and sent me to an endocrinologist who confirmed, after a series of new tests, that I had fibromyalgia and the onset of rheumatoid arthritis. That was another joyous moment in my life. My pain finally had a name. Wow! Now I can be cured! I thought. Then came the shock. They told me there is no cure, just medications to help me manage the symptoms, and that as I age I may even become disabled. I felt like I was standing in court with a judge giving me a sentence: "You are hereby sentenced to a life of pain, misery and heartache. You'll be on medication for the rest of your life. You'll forever be dependent on others as well as a burden. Your life without limits has come to an end!" They told me to exercise—which was a catch 22. I was often in so much pain that it was impossible to exercise, and when I did exercise, I hurt more.

One day my doctor suggested that if I was considering pregnancy, I might find some relief there, as statistics showed that people like me often had permanent change after pregnancy. I wasn't considering pregnancy, but during this time we had a close family friend who had these two adorable kids, Mohit and Arjun. They were loving and authentic. The giving and receiving of unconditional love was amazing. The children were with me so much that people began to think they were mine, which finally got me considering to have my own. When I decided to go ahead, pregnancy was wonderful. I had no pain, my inflammation went away and I lost weight. I had never been happier and I even felt beautiful, something I had never experienced before.

Childbirth was tough though. I ended up having 40 hours of labour. I had preeclampsia, so they had to induce me. I eventually went through an emergency C-Section. However, for the first month everything was great. I couldn't believe I could love anyone so much as I did my son Aman. Then, I started to have symptoms of inflammation and pain to the point that I was bedridden for several months. I was so inflamed I couldn't even hold my baby. I couldn't do anything. There were times when my husband would just put him on the bed beside me so I could feel him and look at him. I couldn't do anything more than that. I finally said this is ridiculous; this is not the way I want to live. I decided I needed to be free from this torment. That was the beginning of my recovery.

So, here is what I learned… When you have a decision to make, always decide without worrying about the how. This is where courage comes into play. You see, in speaking to numerous people in chronic pain I've found they're so used to having a predictable life with support that they begin to enjoy the constant sympathy and attention they receive. As a result, they don't want to change; they're afraid they won't get the same type of love and attention once they are better. I had the same kind of feelings as all the others, but I took the chance anyway. I knew the life of appreciation and courage was far better than sympathy. I've never regretted it. And, now, I'm being recognized for taking action.

At first, it was just Upendra and I. We had family, but they lived far away. My mother had come for two weeks right after I had my baby, but that was it. Upendra was also quite amazing. He was my rock. He would prepare meals for my son and me before going to work, putting the food by my side within reach. I would have to start getting up 45 minutes prior to Aman's feeding. Yes, it would take me 45 minutes of pain, agony and tears to sit up to feed him. I had limited mobility. Upendra would come home and get back to cooking and cleaning. He wouldn't get much time to rest but he never complained or got upset. He was always very optimistic and looked ahead to the future. I guess it was easier for him than for me since he's a visionary guy. Which is why I didn't understand when he started to agree with the doctors that maybe the pain was in my head. Now that I think about it, we had an arranged marriage and had only been married for two years, so he didn't get the chance to know who I really was. We were a work in progress. With all my tests coming back as normal, I guess I would feel that way too. At that time though, I was furious that this thought could even come into his mind.

"The greatest gift of life is friendship, and I have received it."
— **Hubert H. Humphrey**

It was at this time that a close family friend, Mrs. Veena Singla, came on the scene. She was someone who really cared for me regardless of how busy she was with her own family. She also had experience with whole food nutrition. While growing up in India, her family grew their own food, so she had experienced the benefits of farm-to-table concepts, such as fresh fruits and vegetables. She was familiar with the Standard American Diet (SAD) and was also a cancer detection specialist, so she understood the science. In her research for better alternative supplements she'd come across a whole food supplement called Juice Plus. She ordered me to start taking it. I did so because I trusted her, and she was taking it too. However, it was the catalyst the nutritional base, for me to start taking responsibility for my own health. It helped reduce the inflammation and the pain. I was also able to get up and—within four months—start taking care of myself and my baby. This enabled me to make healthier choices. I ate less processed food, did a lot of research and went to a lot of seminars. This opened me up to a whole new community that believed in alternative methods and brought me into contact with people who had similar experiences, confirming to me that it was not all in my head, and that I wasn't crazy. I can't tell you what a relief this was to me. This is when I started to trust myself again. I started to believe that I could live a life without limits. I began to eat less meat and got off wheat, dairy, sugar and processed foods. I was able to exercise on a regular basis, and started working on my mindset.

"When I break the pattern, I break ground. I rebuild when I break down. I wake up more awake than I've been before."
— Pluto

The internal light and the constant voice declaring, "there has to be something better for me" and, "I am meant for so much more" was strong enough that I was able to break the pattern of my behaviour. Today I feel that my son, Aman, was the angel who came to me to make me take the steps I did. You see, doing anything for myself was very difficult. Indian culture is such that the focus is more outward. You are to be giving and caring for members of the family, rather than for yourself. I followed what my mom and grandmother did. I felt caring for my needs was being selfish. I think many women around the globe have felt the same way. Had it not been for the needs of my son, who was born in January of 1998, I wouldn't have taken that first step. I am in gratitude to God and my son for this.

I continued on with my healing journey and found women circles that supported my quest. I noticed a pattern that no matter where I went I always had one or two authentic friends who were there to support me. Whether it was to talk, help with the kids or embark on a girl's night out.

The integration of all of The Four Pillars of Health (nutrition, exercise, mindset and spirituality) has helped me be pain free. On April 27, 2000 when I held my daughter Ashima (my second angel) in my arms for the first time, I wanted her to not be burdened with the generational limitations and beliefs that I had. In order for that to happen I had to change and live differently. This meant overcoming the fears and beliefs I'd carried for several years. It meant breaking the pattern. Ashima inspired me to go even deeper. I wanted our background, culture and challenges to empower my children, to be their strength and foundation. I wanted them to be proud of their 5,000-year heritage. Aman and Ashima have also been great teachers to me. They taught me what unconditional love is. They showed me that they will love me for who I am, even if I don't do anything for them. As I've mentioned, I was taught by my parents that if I didn't do certain things, like getting good grades, then other things would be taken away from me. I was doing the same to my children, I would measure their love by how well they listened to me, but I think they must be old souls because they let me know it didn't have to be that way. You don't have to have one or the other; it's not "or" but "and." Imagine! Loving me just for me! That day I could feel years of built-up walls of shame and heaviness that I had carried all that time melt away. It felt like I lost 30 pounds that day.

It took a long time, but I finally realized all you have to do is begin to care for yourself. You need to show others how to love you by providing them an example through self-love. So often, you do everything for your loved ones, in the hope they'll return the same. But if you don't care for yourself first they'll have no idea as to what you really need in return. Could it be this easy?

By this time, I was hooked on Oprah's "SuperSoul Sunday." I had read several spiritual books by Ekart Tolle, Brene Brown, Elizabeth Lesser and learned how to live a conscious life where you make deliberate choices based on your values and your truth. In doing so, I finally learned that you must be courageous enough to take the first step towards change. As you do this you increase your energetic vibration level and attract like things. As you live better, your vibration increases and you attract similar things within the same vibration level. This is where the saying comes in, "change your thoughts, change your life." For example, those who always think negatively have negative things continue to happen to them. Similarly, those who always think positive, or are optimistic, have more positive things happen to them.

It was with these realizations that I noticed I was attracting more positive, accomplished and heart-centered women who took better care of themselves and their families and were pursuing their passions. I also noticed that I began to release people—even family members—who didn't support me, who were full of negative energy and who drained me of life. I learned that in order to change your life you must be prepared to change the five people you keep company with regularly. You'll find it makes a dramatic difference.

"When people walk away from you, let them go. Your destiny is never tied to anyone who leaves you, and it doesn't mean they are bad people. It just means that their part in your story is over."
— **Tony McCollum**

I started to believe in myself, that I was worthy, and I deserve the best.

"A woman who is convinced that she deserves to accept only the best challenges herself to give the best. Then she is living phenomenally."
— **Maya Angelou**

In 2003 we had the opportunity to go to India. We thought we would go for six months to see if the kids and I would be able to adjust to it. I was excited. I'd always wanted to live in India as an adult, and it was a great time for our kids to get to know our family and culture. Upendra has a big family: six brothers, their spouses, their kids and his extended family. This was scary because I didn't have any close friends or family there. This was an opportunity for us to not only serve our country and the people but also to reconnect with ourselves. Project management was our vehicle to do so. We built our company to 250 employees and trained nearly 100,000 people on project, program and portfolio management. While managing the operation, I trained and counseled professionals on which project management certification would be right for them, based on their years of experience and ambition. I started seeing a pattern of health challenges they were experiencing due to project deadlines and the odd hours required to support global operations. Many had shared that the reason for being in a company or a particular job wasn't because of their passion but because of need. I saw this as a global issue, not just in India. I believe a seed was planted, and I would often think about how I could contribute to people by helping them become healthier and living more fulfilling lives.

As I got to know my in-laws better, I developed a special relationship with my mother-in-law and one particular sister-in-law. Despite the vast differences of our upbringing, my mother-in-law and I connected deeply. She loved me like a son, calling me her seventh son. This is the highest honor she could give me. My sister-in-law's name is Nischal Di. How close are we? Even our birthdays are just a day apart! Nischal Di showed me the parts of myself I'd forgotten. On a regular basis, she would point out my strengths. In all these years, she was the first person who focused on that. She even stood up to my mother when she was not appreciating my successes as I wanted her too. No one had ever done this before. This is when I really started believing in Nischal. Who would take the risk to stand up to a parent if what they were saying wasn't true? In a country where I didn't know anyone, I found a deep authentic connection to someone who believed in me. As a result, the belief that I was meant to contribute in a bigger way was renewed in my heart.

My in-laws had always been progressive and open minded. They made it so easy and comfortable to adapt within the family and in India. The support was amazing and my kids learned the true meaning of a joint family. As a result, we spent ten years in India. It was incredible!

Unfortunately, at the peak of our business, my husband was travelling quite a bit which made it difficult to spend quality time together and the stress of the entrepreneurial roller coaster was so much that old and new symptoms appeared. I had to go back on some medications. During the same time in 2012, my mom was diagnosed with lung cancer. I thought that if my mom, who was so particular about health and diet, could get lung cancer, then anything could be possible with anyone. I was flying back and forth from India to the U.S. for nine months, before moving back to Maryland for the following nine months until she passed away. I was at the peak of my stress—with the uncertainty of my mother's health, the guilt of neglecting my kids and the absence of my husband. It also broke my heart to see my mother suffer. My doctor said I was a prime candidate for a heart attack or a stroke. When my mom died in May 2014, I relocated to Dublin, CA to focus on my health and the children. Over the next two years I was able to rebuild my health.

I've been in business with my husband for over 16 years helping him achieve his dream, and I never really had a connection to myself. I had become an introvert at my parents' hands, and I had followed their plan for me. Then I had been a mother and a businesswoman supporting my husband and his dream. I loved the entrepreneurial journey with my husband. I was able to support him in the way he needed, and I was shaped into a stronger, independent, sharper person thanks to Upendra's habit of throwing me into complex situations and making me fend for myself. Upendra was the blacksmith and I was the iron in the fire getting shaped. I am so thankful to him for that. But I don't think I ever knew myself. So, this is where spirituality really began to work in my life.

> *"Behind every successful woman is a tribe of other successful women who have her back."*
> **— Anonymous**

As I was exploring who I was through the journey of meeting phenomenal women in my community, I attended various seminars and meet-ups. I met a wonderful friend, Becky Diehl, who runs a forgiveness ministry with her husband Steve. Becky and Steve have been instrumental in helping me understand what forgiveness means. Although their program is bible based, I was still able to understand. Becky explained the message of God in a simple, practical manner that applied to today's life. This deepened my spiritual insights. She helped me reconnect with Hinduism and I truly began to understand the concept of God within myself. In fact, I can say through Jesus I was able to understand and connect to Hinduism better. This is a true integration of community and culture. I also began to listen to transformational leaders and coaches like Tony Robbins, Jim Rohn and The Secret team. One day when I was listening to Lisa Nichols, I learned why I needed to share my story. She said when you go through a major life challenge or solve a complex problem, the story is not yours to keep. You must share. You don't have to be a victim. You can change the meaning to be something that helps others—by telling your story.

> *"Always look at the solution, not the problem. Learn to focus on what will give results."*
> **— Anonymous**

The question in your mind right now must be what is the real solution? I believe this is going to be an ongoing exploration. Here are some suggestions to get you started. You'll need to keep in mind that everyone is unique and has specific needs. The key is to pay attention to what works for you. How well you do will depend on your commitment to practice.

- Look at holistic integrated healing. Our body is an integrated machine, and what happens in one area affects another. Holistic inquiry is to establish the root cause instead of just treating the

117

symptoms. Sure, the medical community is crucial in our healing journey. But, we need to work as partners and be proactive rather than reactive. Functional medicine seems to address this philosophy. Find a doctor who shares your values and health philosophy. Ask lots of questions of your medical care team, and don't be afraid to get multiple opinions.

- Try an elimination diet. Start with eliminating gluten, dairy and red meat.

- Follow a clean diet. Add as many raw vegetables as you can. Eat organic as much as you can. You can even become an urban gardener, like me, and grow your vegetables on your balcony.

- Make sure your plumbing is working properly. It is important that you are expelling waste properly and regularly, both urinating and excreting. This is especially important before you detox. This happens when your gut is clean. Not passing waste is like not cleaning your fish bowl for months. Yes, it's really bad.

- Exercise consistently. What is the best form of exercise? The one you will do. The idea is to move your body. So do your favorite activity.

- Allocate sufficient time for sleep. This is when your body restores and recharges.

- Have the courage to listen to your inner compass and follow its guidance. Trust your gut and listen to your heart.

- Practice Daily Self-care and Self-love. This includes giving yourself permission to breakdown and cry

- Release emotions that no longer serve you. Open up space for new experiences to enter.

- Process unprocessed emotions. Let go and forgive.

- Ask for help. You're still a strong, respectable person, even if you ask for help.

- Stand up for yourself and make your voice be heard. This doesn't mean you have to be aggressive or put anyone else down. It does mean paying attention to your likes and dislikes.

- Reduce your stress. It's important to understand what triggers your stress and your flare-ups. When you know them, then you can actively remove them or avoid them. For a free assessment on How to Identify Your Trigger Points write to me at seema@seemagiri. com.

- Be in action!

It sounds like a lot of work doesn't it? To be honest it is, but it's so worth it! Right now you may not even believe that you can do this. It may feel overwhelming. I get it. I felt that way too. But the reality is that if you don't try, you'll never be able to do it. In fact, the very reason you should be doing this is because you don't believe in yourself enough to be convinced it will work. When you engage, you'll greatly change your confidence. The areas you resist the most are the greatest growth areas. Everyday that goes by where you don't engage in taking action towards improving your health, you're letting one more day pass you by that could have been more awesome. You might not care now, but consider this: as you lay on your deathbed and you review your life, the only things you'll regret aren't the shots you took and missed but the shots you never took that could have made your time on earth more magnificent. Not to mention that your family depends on you to make the changes that both you and they need. What legacy do you want to leave behind?

As Theodore Roosevelt says, "Do what you can from where you are with what you have!" This is actually a spiritual practice. Like Nike's slogan, "Just do it!" done consistently.

Life is not supposed to be difficult. You can get through it with ease and grace. The challenges we encounter are really there to teach us a lesson or sharpen us even more. If you stay true to your nature, life is easier and things start to fall into place effortlessly. The best analogy is that we are diamonds in the rough. The challenges are supposed to polish us so we can shine with our light; with the gift we're supposed to bring into this world. I truly believe that all of us have a unique purpose in life that is meant to be shared.

"The best way to get rid of the pain is to feel the pain. And when you feel the pain and go beyond it, you'll see there's a very intense love that is wanting to awaken itself."
— **Deepak Chopra**

Believe it or not, I consider my autoimmune disease a blessing in disguise. It forced me to reclaim my nature and voice in this lifetime, while I can still make a difference in the world. Today I'm a successful businesswoman, involved mother, supportive wife and active community member. I serve as a board member and I perform leadership roles in non-profits in my community. It gave me the opportunity to connect the dots and let me reconnect to myself in a profound way. It has also enabled me to connect more deeply and authentically with my children, husband and friends. I have thriving relationships. I'm pain free and off of 25 medications. I am down to only one and even for that, the dosage is reduced. I'm still making dietary changes. From time to time I get off my healthy track and indulge in sinful pleasures such as chocolate and ice cream. I simply get back on track without beating myself up and without judgement. I'm still learning. I'm a work in progress. Most importantly, I've found my purpose and passion. My life's work is to help women with autoimmune disease or symptoms, through …

- Personal, loving coaching to build your confidence and courage, and walk beside you through your recovery journey.

- Bridging the gap between your doctor's allopathic care and mind-body-spirit practices to create a holistic recovery plan.

- Advocating for you with your doctors and caregivers; work with your family to support you in your journey to a new life.

"The moment a woman decides to be unafraid she is transformed. When she recognizes the power and possibilities of her own strength and surrenders every fear to that power, she becomes the greatest version of herself."
— **Diane Von Furstenberg**

What can I do for you? As Denis Waitley says, "Time and Health are the two most precious assets that we don't recognize and appreciate until they have been depleted." The thing that bothered me the most was the time I lost being controlled by and managing my pain; time lost with family, time lost with my son and time lost where I didn't make a financial contribution to the family. While I can't recover that time, it has taught me to be more present and cherish every moment. This is my invitation to you to get your health and your time back, to design a life that brings you more control, energy, and balance. My work addresses the whole you—body-mind-spirit—and is drawn from the best practices in holistic healing, ancient eastern modalities, my own "kitchen-tested" practices and love. I want to hold your hand while you embark on your own journey of self-discovery—in the way only someone who has walked the path can. I've developed a program called "Take Charge of Your Health Blueprint for Women with Autoimmune Disease," which includes the strategies and life hacks I've created over the years. In this program you'll learn how to nourish your body and soul, how to energize yourself and how to take massive action and measure yourself based on your beliefs and standards. The point is to create simple systems that will help create a structure in your life that's specific to your needs.

My questions to you: Are you ready to break free from your pain cycle and TAKE BACK YOUR POWER? If you are ready to take charge of your recovery, then please contact me to schedule a free 30-minute Take Charge Session at seema@seemagiri.com

> *"There is no greater gift you can receive than to honor your calling.*
> *It's why you were born and how you become most truly alive."*
> **— Oprah Winfrey**

Thank You!

Find Your True Self with Yoga and Pole

LYNNE NIEPAGE

A few years ago, I visited Las Vegas for a NASCAR event. One evening my friend's brother drove a group of us in his car to meet their aunt for dinner. I twisted around in the front seat so I could better see my friends in the back seat and chatted excitedly when we were stopped at a stoplight. We were at the stoplight on Flamingo Road heading away from the Las Vegas Strip when an underage, impaired driver hit us doing between 60-70 mph.

The impact on the rear driver's side pushed us forward about one and a half car lengths. It sounded like a bomb had gone off and debris flew everywhere as the driver bounced off a Mustang convertible beside us and went airborne over us. Yes, I saw the whole underside of his car as it went over us. There was axle grease up the side of our car!

The impaired driver was taken away by ambulance; he survived the accident and we heard he eventually ended up skipping the country to avoid prosecution. Some witnesses stopped after the accident and waited with us until the investigator arrived. They said the driver who hit us was passed out in his car at a previous stoplight. I do not know if someone honked at him causing him to slam his foot on the accelerator before passing out again or just what happened. The investigator said the driver never even put on the brakes before hitting us!

The post-accident debris field was probably 100 square feet or more, leaving five lanes closed for about three hours. First the firemen arrived, then the paramedics, then the police, followed by the investigator. Finally, the flatbeds came to remove our car and the drunk's car (the Mustang was still drivable).

I was happy and rather amazed that I was alive and basically intact, but I never did make it to NASCAR. Shock is a funny thing. I recall saying to the girl in the Mustang, "Aren't you glad the Mustang convertible was the first convertible ever to receive the 5 Star crash safety rating?"

Unfortunately, since I was twisted in my seat when the accident occurred, I ended up with a protruded lumbar disc, a concussion, a dent in my skull, and whiplash. The following months were filled with brain and back doctors, a chiropractor, imaging, and epidural injections. But me being the typical female, I was worried about the ever-increasing size of my butt. You see, I have less than stellar eating habits (I like tasty food), and in the past, I had used running to burn calories so I could eat the foods I like. With the damage to my spine, running was not only painful but not advised. Of course, it was a vicious circle because the more weight I gained from lack of exercise, the more my back hurt which made exercise more painful.

I decided to find something new and low-impact that would keep me interested so that I would stick with it long enough to make a positive difference in my body. I decided to try pole dancing. I mean, doesn't everyone? It piqued my interest and it looked fun, so I decided to give it a try. I went online to find a local studio and signed up for a class.

My trial class was the following Saturday. I awoke that morning excited and a little anxious. Would my back be able to handle pole dancing? Would I look stupid doing it? Would everyone else be better than me? Would I even like it?

Would I stick with it?

I squared my shoulders, gave myself a pep talk, and headed out. The class began with introductions and, happily for me, with gentle stretches and moves to warm up the spine and body. When the instructor ended the class, I was surprised it was over. Time had flown by and I felt great! I was surprised that I not only felt better physically, but I felt better emotionally too. I was hooked!

After that first class, I convinced my friend, who had been in the car accident with me, to sign up for the next session. It was enlightening to discover that we both enjoyed the class even though our body types are very different. Some things came easier to me and some were easier for her, but we both saw improvements in ourselves. I have since learned that this is an experience that opens your eyes to each individual's unique beauty. Every person in the class is on their own journey, each different, but we all share a supportive experience.

The more I attended classes over the following months, the better and stronger I felt. As I progressed, my core strengthened and I became more flexible which, as it turns out, was incredibly good for my back. I always left the studio feeling better than when I arrived. I now refer to it as Pole Therapy!

JUST4MIE

I received a job transfer back home with my day job and decided to open my own studio. That is how Just4MiE was born! Contrary to the beliefs of some, this kind of pole dancing empowers women. When you take a pole dancing class, your mind and body stretch and develop. You will learn to respect your body's strengths and appreciate your own unique beauty as you gain confidence and self-worth. I created Just4MiE for every woman, no matter her age, shape, size, or fitness level. My desire is that every woman experience the joy and satisfaction I felt after my first class.

After several years and a flood (yes, flood, but that is another story), I decided that I did not want to pay an unresponsive landlord the high ticket rent anymore. So, I developed a plan. My lease was up for renewal the following spring and they required six months' notice if I planned to cancel. It was summer, so that only gave me a few months to put my plan in motion.

I was going to sell my house and buy a live/work building where I could have the studio in the commercial space and live above it. I would be close to the studio; my entire commute would be down a set of stairs. It was brilliant! The only obstacle left was to find one.

It turns out that finding a live/work unit in the right location with suitable ceiling height and layout (both studio and home) was harder than I expected. I finally found a new build that would work. It was perfect and the close date matched up with the last month at the current studio!

Unfortunately, I was twentieth in line and they were sold before my turn came up. Not to be deterred, I awaited the next release and made sure I did not miss out this time by sleeping in the parking lot the night before the release! Even showing up at noon the day before the release I was twenty-sixth in line and there were only ten units available. Of those ten, only four were suitable for a studio and only two had the layout I wanted.

The drill was to check in every four hours to keep your place in line, but I and many others were not going to take the chance of missing roll call, so we set up camp in the parking lot! Roll call after roll call the numbers dwindled. At the nine o'clock AM opening I was in sixth position. I got my unit of choice!

The close date meant I would be closed for three months, which was not ideal, but I was happy to have what would become the new studio. The last newly-built home I purchased had no construction delays, so I was not prepared for what ended up being a sixteen-month delay!

When the first delay occurred, I reached out to a fellow studio owner to see if she minded that I take classes at her studio so I could keep dancing. Turns out, she did mind. Then my sister suggested yoga and I agreed it was a perfect idea. So, I used the construction delays to get my yoga teaching certification.

Yoga is the perfect complement to pole dancing! Both get you to pay attention to your movement, physical and mental balance, mindfulness, breathing, strength, and flexibility. Adding aerial yoga, as well, gives you a natural progression from the earth to the air!

At Just4MiE I decided to offer yoga classes along with pole dance classes; therefore, the operating name had to change. Yoga and Pole™ was born! The health benefits of yoga are well-known and extensive. Yoga not only increases flexibility and builds muscle, but it also can do the following when practiced regularly: lower blood pressure, improve bone health, increase blood flow, improve sleep, balance, and focus, among many additional benefits.

Pole dance and yoga complement each other well. In pole dancing you will use muscles you may not have known you had! I have yoga classes that are designed specifically to stretch and strengthen muscles used in my pole dance classes. I also incorporate yoga in my pole dance classes via the warm-up, breathing technique while holding poses, and the cool down. The combination of grounding meditation and yoga, the sassy fun of sensual dance, and the strength-building of moves on the pole ensure a uniquely fun way to be active and build confidence. It is the workout that does not feel like work!

If you are unfamiliar with the concept of pole fitness, you may be a bit shocked by the idea. Pole-dancing often gets a bad rap but it is time to stop associating pole dance with stripping. Pole dance is a complete workout that combines cardiovascular fitness with resistance training and flexibility. You will be impressed as you witness changes in your strength, grace, and, yes, sensuality. You can soon be in the best shape of your life!

Many people think the only reason to learn pole-dancing is to perform for others. So wrong! The women who attend my classes do so for themselves. It is empowering and improves your self-image, which is a positive thing. If you happen to share what you have learned, it is a gift not a requirement!

Just4MiE's studio is designed for the comfort of my clients. In the beginning, some women are uncomfortable with themselves and worry about seeing their jiggly bits in the mirror, so I offer to cover the mirrors. I want women to focus on how they feel on the inside, not how they look on the outside. My clients learn to focus on their form by listening to my voice and feeling the movement in their body rather than focusing on what they see in the mirror.

Soon they begin seeing themselves differently as their body image changes. They no longer notice their jiggly bits; they notice a strong, confident woman who is willing to work hard to feel better inside and out. While working on the outside, I also encourage women to work on the inside by challenging their limiting beliefs about themselves.

A limiting belief is any idea or belief you hold to be true that holds you back in some way. We all have them, but some of us never acknowledge them. Once acknowledged, a limiting belief can be challenged and eradicated. This may sound simple, but it is not as easy as it sounds.

Pay attention to what you say to yourself through the day. Is it something you would say to the person sitting next to you? If not, do not say it to yourself. Is it mostly positive or mostly negative? For every negative thought, substitute a positive one. The longest relationship you will ever have in your life is with yourself. Make it a great relationship! Be kind to yourself.

When I think of limiting beliefs, Beverly comes to mind. She was practically dragged to a trial class by a friend. Beverly was not an ideal weight when I first met her but, more importantly, she did not believe she deserved to feel good about herself. At the beginning of a trial class there are often nervous giggles, but Beverly did not crack a smile. By the end of class, she had relaxed and seemed to be enjoying herself. I was thrilled when she signed up and continued to attend regularly.

By practicing meditation along with physical fitness Beverly became aware of the limiting beliefs she had about herself and began to challenge them. She tuned in to her inner dialogue and realized just how hostile she was to herself. She began to change her inner dialogue by giving herself grace and learning to be kind to herself.

Beverly has since lost weight and toned up; now she likes how she looks on the outside. However, she loves the confident woman she has become on the inside! The limiting belief that she is not deserving still pops in from time to time, but she is now aware of these negative thoughts and does not allow them to remain for long.

MARCIE

Marcie is one of the most beautiful people you can imagine. Her angelic looks and amazingly fit body make you think she must have some tragic flaw in her personality to balance it all out. But you would be wrong; she also has a very sweet, selfless nature and goes out of her way to help others.

One summer evening, Marcie first came to the studio for a bachelorette party. Afterward, she asked me about the timing of the first session of the next year since she had commitments that would prevent her from attending the fall sessions. Typically, when someone puts off starting a session, I don't expect to see them again but that did not happen with Marcie. Come the new year, she was there and thereafter attended weekly for years!

As I got to know her, I realized Marcie did not see herself as I, or others, saw her. Through months of classes, I saw her become more comfortable with her body and her femininity. I still remember the joyous expression on her face when she completed one of her special assignment graduation dances; she had finally gotten outside of her head and danced her emotions!

This was also an important reminder for me that what is going on outside of a person is not always a reflection of what is happening on the inside. Each person's journey is different and relative to their own true self, not to yours.

Dancing to what you feel and relating to the music instead of thinking about what you look like or what others will think is truly liberating! It can allow you to release painful or negative emotions and, conversely, it can amplify happy, joyous emotions. We have methods for helping you achieve this liberation, but I will not divulge those secrets here. (The "liberating" is referring to your mind and emotions, not body parts, as there is never any nudity in the studio!)

It is natural when you are in a supportive environment like our studio to feel comfortable sharing deeper emotions and life experiences than you ever would at the local gym! The studio is like Vegas; what happens in the studio, stays in the studio!

IT IS A PROCESS

Another student, Jan, taught me a valuable lesson. When a competition organizer came to the studio and asked if I had any students that would be competing in the upcoming pole dance weekend, I responded that I would post the flyer, but I doubted that any students would compete.

I was projecting my limiting belief onto my students. I did not like to be the center of attention and assumed that my students would not be interested in competing until they had mastered the sport. When I mentioned the competition to some students, Jan did show a hint of interest. Luckily, I realized my mistake and fully supported her preparation for the competition.

I am so grateful that I did not let my fears get in the way of supporting Jan and her entry into the competition. Yes, she did get a medal in her category but that is not the point. Her dance was so beautiful and very moving; it reminded me how important the emotional component is in dance and that you should not hold back just because you are "in process." I thank Jan for reminding me of that!

We have a tough time being "in process." We want to make changes and have the results yesterday! We have difficulty settling for anything less than perfection, which starts the cycle of self-doubt when we are human and do not master change on the first (or second, or tenth) try. We are usually our own worst critics too. We often feel that we must master a move, skill, or task before we can be happy with ourselves. This is not true! Be content to be in process; do not wait for the final accomplishment to feel your joy. Be proud of each step you take towards your goal!

I am sure you have seen one of those picture progressions showing what the model really looked like followed by the filtered lenses and Photoshop steps needed to get the final advertisement. Or I know you have seen a twenty-year-old model demonstrating the benefits of an anti-wrinkle cream in the pages of a magazine. How about the pudgy, pale, sad guy who develops muscles and a tan in 'just four weeks' by trying the latest diet and exercise fad? It is no surprise that we are rarely successful when we try to get the advertised results immediately upon using the product or service. It should come as no surprise that you may feel inadequate when you see your image in a mirror; you are comparing yourself to something that does not even exist in nature!

I think that there should be truth in advertising to the degree that only people who use the product or service advertise it. Do not get me wrong, I am all about aspiring to be the best you can be. I just think the image of what that is should be realistic!

There is no "one size fits all" self-improvement plan because we are all unique. We each have unique body shapes and contours, facial features, life experiences, and genetics; we all have our own unique beauty. Let your unique beauty shine!

Nothing is more attractive than a woman who is confident and comfortable with who she is. I lost my confidence after my car accident. Not being able to run took a mental toll just as it took a physical one. I missed those endorphins! I missed feeling good after a hard workout!

Words cannot express how much my life has improved since I tried that first pole dance class. Learning to do something physically challenging that I never dreamed I could do was incredibly empowering. Obviously, I am passionate about pole fitness and yoga because I opened my own studio and now share my love with others. If you would like to find a Yoga and Pole™ in your neighborhood, check my website Yoga and Pole™ for a location where you will always get the special intimacy you feel at the friendly neighborhood studio and where you will find your true self! If you are considering opening your own studio, contact me for Yoga and Pole™ franchise information.

During a Yoga and Pole™ by Just4MiE class you will you will meet and make new friends while participating in a meditation and a workout which can include yoga, dance, and/or pole! I would love for you to join me! If you cannot get to Yoga and Pole™ in your neighborhood, my advice is to try a few different studios and instructors in your area to find the best fit for you. Visit my website, www.yogaandpole.com, then sign up for my newsletter at http://bit.ly/2ueMUoT.

The Modern Healer

HERMAN SIU
& MARTIN SIU

ood health is a God-given right; it's our birthright. Yet, while we
have made huge technological advances to facilitate cross-planet
communication in real-time, we haven't been as progressive in
keeping ourselves healthy.

We may be living longer but, tragically, children are dying from cancers,
diabetes is on the rise, and young adults are suddenly getting heart attacks.
Chronic fatigue, depression, and anxiety assail us. We rely on drugs to fix our
health problems and we spend billions of dollars on prescriptions that may
alleviate the symptoms but leave the root cause untouched. In our fast-paced
societies, we have lost the connection with nature and the natural elements
that make up our bodies. Surely, there is an alternative way to heal ourselves,
or even to prevent disease from occurring in the first place.

The long and short of it is that we don't have to drop out of society and reside in the woods to live happier and healthier lives. The answer to good health and longevity lies right at our fingertips – in the air we breathe, the foods we eat, and water we drink. That's the best prescription for the Modern Healer, and these are the guiding principles we use in our healing practice. As 5th and 6th generation healers immersed in traditions that date back to ancient Chinese Shaolin practices, we adhere to the disciplined and holistic approach of our forefathers.

We believe that a body in full balance has everything it needs to fight off disease, stay and look young, and be active and involved, regardless of the biological age. This belief has been supported by patient outcomes through successive centuries of practice by the healers in our family. We share this knowledge with you to empower you as a Modern Healer, so that you may take control of and assume responsibility for your own health and be the expert in your own healing and wellness journey.

To be empowered as a Modern Healer, you must first understand the core concepts of energy or Qi (chi) as defined by ancient Chinese healing texts.

Dr. Paul Unschuld, a highly-regarded authority on Chinese medicine and multi-book author said, "The core Chinese concept of qi bears no resemblance to the Western concept of 'energy'. We perceive that there is a knowledge gap in the current understanding of eastern medicine in the western world. Mindful of the wisdom suggested by the Chinese proverb, "A journey of a thousand miles begins with a single step," we have written this chapter as our first step towards bridging that divide.

There are three primary components to balance Qi. Qi is a fundamental power underlying all of nature, and it is a vital life force that runs through our body. There are three primary components to balance our Qi. The first component to boosting our Qi is the air we breathe, the second is the food we eat, and the third is the water we drink.

AIR GIVES LIFE

Almost all of life needs oxygen to survive. We take in oxygen from our surroundings to harness energy and use it to power the inner workings of our bodies.

In the Huangdi Neijing, the ancient Chinese foundation medical text, the lungs breathe in what's known as, da qi, or "great qi.". Once we breathe in the air, the lungs extract the Qi from the da qi. Based on this understanding, we perceive that Qi relates to life-sustaining oxygen.

What is the secret to having great Qi? It is the harmonization of the mind, body, and spirit.

In martial arts, we use our mind to harness Qi by controlling our breath. We use our body to breathe, and we put our bodies through constant practice to master our Qi. Once it has been mastered, the Qi can be at our fingertips in a moment's notice. We call it in this form the spirit.

Viewed from this perspective, it's simple to make the most of living and get the best use of your life. The first step to taking back control of your health is by learning to breathe correctly.

Notice, right this moment, how you are breathing. Are you breathing from your diaphragm or the stomach, or are you taking in quick snatches of air? The majority of us take shallow breaths because we have forgotten how to breathe deeply and fully, and the only time we do so is when we are in yoga or meditation. Having become a society of superficial breathers, we are not benefitting from the fact that 70% of the toxins in our bodies are released through breath. By breathing shallowly, we are shortchanging ourselves because hypoxia, or insufficient oxygen in the body's cells, has been linked to degenerative diseases.

Remember, breath equals life and a long breath enhances a long life. Breathing correctly is your first responsibility as a Modern Healer.

FOOD FOR HEALING

The second primary component to balance our Qi is food.

The ancient Greek physician, Hippocrates, who is widely known as the "Father of Medicine", is quoted as saying "Let food be thy medicine and medicine be thy food." Fast forward several centuries; Dr. Roger J. Williams, who discovered the B-vitamin, said in 1971, "The human body heals itself and nutrition provides the resources to accomplish the task." The Chinese are well known to eat their food in its season. For example, no watermelon is eaten in winter since it grows in the hot summer climate.

It is empowering to discover that we need look no further than our own gardens and our kitchens to find healing nutrition that supports health for our family. By making healthy food choices, we ensure that we age gracefully and live out the rest of the twilight years harmoniously and peacefully, without the blight of Alzheimer's, dementia, or other failing diseases.

"So many people spend their health gaining wealth & then have to spend their wealth to regain their health." - Chinese proverb

Our philosophy is that, with right air, right food and right water (in this order), you detoxify naturally, without having to go on rigid short-term fasts.

With the right balance of foods that are appropriate to your body type, you'll get rid of excess fat and flab, find the correct body weight, be brimming over with energy, have the mental clarity to solve challenges with ease, and be in love with your life.

If you're tired of feeling frustrated, angry, depressed, unsure, overweight, tired, and in despair, look to your shopping list, refrigerator and kitchen closets for the culprits. Are they full of processed foods and refined sugars? Are you eating natural grains, green leafy vegetables and fresh fruit?

In this chapter, we'll draw on healing secrets that we share with our clients in our Toronto-based clinic. We'll discuss the major foods that prevent inflammation, help you recover from cuts and wounds, and help detoxify the system.

But for the Modern Healer, the first line of defense is maintaining a healthy pH balance. Acid is corrosive and is the biggest culprit of many degenerative and deadly diseases. It's true that some acid is needed in the body. The stomach uses it to break down the food we eat into macronutrients such as proteins, fats and carbohydrates, and micronutrients such as vitamins and minerals that it may be easily absorbed by the body. But most typical diets are packed with sugar, animal proteins, and processed foods.

WHY PH BALANCE IS CRUCIAL TO GOOD HEALTH

The pH is a measure of acidity or alkalinity. The billions of cells that make up our bodies need an alkaline environment to function, to stay healthy, and to regenerate. Too much acid in our bodies creates ripe conditions for the growth of bacteria, yeast, fungus, viruses, mold and other diseases. Cells that are starved of oxygen are unable to regenerate. Once starved, they are unable to repair damage or rid the body of noxious chemicals and toxins. In time, the cells die; research now points out that cancer is the result of an over-acidic body. An ideal balance for our bodies is measured between a pH of 7.2 – 7.4. You can measure this by dipping pH testing strips into a sample of saliva or urine. An acidic body will produce a pH reading of less than 7.2, which means there is a lack of oxygenation at the cellular level. Your body may even create more fat cells to store the corrosive acid, leading to unwanted weight gain. If the body is malnourished or lacking any Alkaline minerals, it goes in search of calcium to optimize the pH level, and extracts calcium from your bones (joints), teeth and tissues which in turn leaves the bones weak. Calcium is one of the most important alkaline minerals as it increases the oxygen level in the blood. This calcium depletion results in arthritis and osteoporosis. In the initial stages of over-acidity, you may suffer from joint pains, headaches, and weight gain. In an acidic state, the body is trying to expel excess acid through your skin, causing muscle cramps, eczema, acne, swelling, irritation, and general aches and pains. People in this state get grouchier and irritable, and they age faster than those with a balanced pH body. Other so-called modern diseases linked to an acidic body include diabetes, osteoarthritis, acid reflux, irritable bowel syndrome, premature aging, muscle and chronic fatigue, bone loss and osteoporosis.

"The only way to keep good health is to eat what you don't want, drink what you don't like, & do what you'd rather not" -Chinese proverb

GETTING YOUR PH BALANCE RIGHT THROUGH FOODS

Our experience has shown that a balanced diet should be 85-90% alkaline and 10-15% acidic. Body functions and hand-eye coordination work at their optimal state at these levels. It's better for the body to be slightly alkaline than it is to be slightly acidic. Now that we understand why the pH balance is the first line of defense and why it's crucial to maintain the correct pH balance, let's explore quickly what foods contribute to a more alkaline state and more acidic state. A food is classified as alkaline or acidic according to its mineral content. Alkaline-forming foods contain more minerals such as calcium, magnesium, manganese, iron, and potassium. Some acid-promoting minerals include phosphorous, copper, and sulfur. Carbonated drinks are acid forming because they are loaded with sugar and phosphorus, which can lead to weight gain. Have a healthy serving of kale or broccoli instead, which nourishes your body with helpful calcium and magnesium for bone and muscle health. Alkaline foods include apples, apricots, cantaloupes, cauliflower, broccoli, kale, almonds, chestnuts and walnuts. The complete list is much longer and we will examine the healing qualities of alkaline-based nutrition in the section under Anti-Inflammation Foods. Acidic foods include ice-cream, manufactured processed foods with refined sugar, meat, fish, poultry, and eggs. This is not to say that all fruits and vegetables are alkaline. Some are in fact very acidic. Acidic vegetables include corn, onions, and garlic. In the fruit category will fall cranberries, blueberries, and currants. As you grow older, it's harder to expel the acid that is in your body. The longer acid exists, the more it will congeal and the more it will attack your cells and immune system. Acidic conditions manifest one illness at a time. Symptoms include arthritis, muscle fatigue, and body aches. At the point that you are weakest is when you're most prone to infections and diseases because infections live off acidic waste products. At our clinic, we will examine the root cause of your health problems, not just the symptoms. We will customize a holistic healing plan drawing on our experience and expertise to restore you to the right balance, homeostasis, so you may live your life in joy and harmony.

"Tell me and I'll forget; show me and I may remember; involve me and I'll understand" - Chinese proverb

ALKALINE AND ANTI-INFLAMMATION FOODS

Inflammation is a natural body response to injury. You bruise when you hit your shin against a table leg or when you sprain an ankle. Chronic inflammation, if undetected, can result in debilitating illnesses such as heart disease, cancer, diabetes, arthritis, and Alzheimer's. Fried and processed foods, as well as foods that contain trans-fat, increase the risk of inflammation. We've mentioned that alkaline foods prevent inflammation, and these are ordinary fruits, vegetables, and herbs that you can find in your refrigerator, spice cabinet, and even in your own garden. There are many creative ways to prepare these foods for a delicious, nutritious, beneficial anti-inflammation diet/alkaline diet. Here is a small list of foods to keep your body in balance and in good health.

Avocados: they contain healthy fats, phyto-proteins, vitamins, minerals and dietary fiber that is sorely lacking in the western societies. Low in sugar content, avocados may help to lower cholesterol levels, and increase resistance to diabetes, coronary heart disease, stroke and cancer, while promoting a healthy body weight and body mass index (BMI). Avocados are best eaten fresh.

Bamboo shoots: which is not a common vegetable on the western table, were identified by the Compendium of Materia Medica, the most comprehensive medical book in the history of traditional Chinese Medicine. Bamboo shoots promote the circulatory system, supplementing the body's natural energy, and are recommended as a daily dish. A traditional forest vegetable in Chinese diets for 2,500 years, nutrient-rich bamboo shoots are being shown in modern research to help prevent cancer, and to aid in weight loss, digestion, and the appetite.

Bamboo shoots are rich in essential amino acids and fatty acids and, because of their low sugar content, they are useful for treating hypertension, hyperlipemia, and hyperglycemia.

Broccoli: just about all vegetables are good, but some are more alkaline than others. Broccoli counts among the latter as it is rich in important vitamins such as A, C, K, B-complex and minerals including iron, zinc, and phosphorus. Broccoli is also rich in phytonutrients, which are natural chemicals that help protect plants and prevent disease in our bodies.

Broccoli helps to prevent osteoarthritis, reduces the risk of cancer, and has been shown to help reverse diabetes and heart damage. Broccoli is best lightly steamed or gently stir-fried; overcooking will neutralize its benefits.

Cabbage: A source of Vitamins K, C, B6, folate, and thiamine. Cabbage is also a source of iodine to support the health of the brain and the nervous system. This vegetable, which is a staple in Chinese kitchens around the world, helps to lower cholesterol and is rich in glucosinolates that are shown to have cancer prevention properties.

Carrot: Raw or cooked, carrots are a rich source of Vitamins A and C, calcium and iron, and the anti-oxidant beta-carotene that gives the vegetable its orange colour. In addition, carrots contain fibre, Vitamins K and E, potassium, folate, manganese, magnesium, zinc, and some phosphorus. Carrots improve our vision, delay aging, help with regulating blood sugar, improve digestion, and help prevent cancer. There is a side note to add: overconsumption of carrots can be toxic so, if you start turning orange, you may want to cut back on your carrot intake!

Cauliflower: The cauliflower is packed with vitamins such as B1, B2, B3,

B5, B6, B9, C and K, as well as being rich in omega 3, fatty acids, fibre, manganese, and potassium. Apart from delivering powerful antioxidants, cauliflower is a healthy source of protein and fibre, it enhances the body's ability to detoxify, reduces the risk of inflammation and the incidence of cancer. Cauliflower is best lightly cooked through a simple sauté.

Spinach: Spinach is widely acknowledged to be rich in vitamins and minerals such as magnesium, iron, copper, calcium, potassium, and zinc. The dark green spinach is packed with anti-oxidants and health-promoting phyto-nutrients. If you're low in iron, spinach helps to make up the deficit. It is an aid in the management of diabetes, and works towards lowering high blood pressure and improving bone health. Spinach is best eaten lightly steamed, quickly boiled or sautéed.

Ginger: Mankind's historic cure-all, ginger is rich in anti-oxidants, vitamins and minerals, and also contains omega-3 and omega-6. Shown to be anti-inflammatory, anti-cancer, anti-nausea, and a powerful anti-oxidant, it greatly boosts the immune system. A versatile root, ginger can be chewed fresh, steamed, boiled in water to make tea, or grated and added to sautéed dishes.

The state in which it is consumed will affect its benefits greatly. Fresh ginger root fights the common cold, coughs, and asthma, while dried ginger root is better against abdominal pain, cold limbs, and rheumatism. If you were to use the fresh root for rheumatism, the condition will worsen but, fresh or dried, it is effective in preventing or stopping vomiting and diarrhea. Large quantities of fresh ginger are not recommended for those with high blood pressure, inflammatory bowel disease, ulcers, or intestinal blockage, and should be used sparingly if you suffer from gallstones. Excessive consumption can cause a person to break out in a rash as an allergic reaction and may also lead to heartburn, bloating, gas, belching, and even some nausea. From ginger root, we'll move on to alkaline-forming fruit and herbs to round up our short list of recommended foods. Remember, some foods are mildly acidic and some are weak acidic foods. Not all acidic foods are tarred with the same brush, but the worst offenders include processed foods, sugar, tomatoes, onions, garlic, dairy, and vinegar.

Apricot: the fruit and the seeds are effective alkaline-forming foods. Packed with iron and protein, apricots are good for quenching thirst and fighting asthma. The seeds from the bitter apricot heal coughs, sore throats, and constipation, as does the sweet apricot seed. But those suffering from asthma should eat only the bitter apricot seed, or the condition will worsen. Laetrile, a naturally occurring substance found in the kernels, has been increasingly promoted to help in cancer treatment. The apricot kernels have been documented to help fight against tumors as far back as 502 AD. The apricot oil has been used as far back as 17th century England to fight swellings, tumors, and ulcers

Peppermint: a herb with healing benefits dating back to ten thousand years in the past, peppermint is commonly used to fight inflammation. It soothes abdominal pain, indigestion, irritable bowels and bloating, and prevents nausea and vomiting. It is a popular healing food for the common colds that are accompanied by headaches, sore throat and thick phlegm. However, if you are suffering a common cold but have a runny nose, cold limbs and diarrhea, peppermint is not that effective. Although it is commonly thought of as an herb or a spice, it is actually cool and pungent, and should not be used daily. Those suffering from anemia or low blood pressure should use only as directed.

"Health is the greatest gift, Contentment is the greatest treasure, Confidence is the greatest friend, Enlightenment is the greatest bliss." -Chinese proverb

FOODS TO ACCELERATE HEALING OF CUTS AND WOUNDS

Skin is the biggest organ in our bodies, and we tend to take it for granted because small nicks heal quickly. However, there are times when there is a deep cut or wound from an accident or from surgery when extra support is required for the connective tissue to regenerate. Connective tissue is different from most other tissues because it is made not so much of cells, but from protein, notably collagen, fibres encased in a unique covering called a fascia. To boost your ability to heal quickly from cuts and wounds, look for foods with these four pivotal nutrients and minerals.

Vitamin C: Vitamin C assists in forming collagen to repair the connective tissue in the blood vessels, cartilage, muscles, and in the bones. Good sources of Vitamin C include fruits such as guava, kiwi, strawberries, and papaya. Vegetables include red and green sweet peppers, Brussels sprouts, broccoli, cauliflower, and sweet potatoes.

Vitamin A: Some of the foods mentioned in the category above will be useful for sourcing Vitamin A because they are rich beta-carotene that is converted into fully active Vitamin A. This vitamin serves many functions. It promotes growth, maintains the immune system, and supports vision. Other Vitamin A rich foods are sweet potatoes, pumpkins, carrots, spinach, turnip greens, and cantaloupe.

Flavonoids: These are a group of pigments that give plants their colour but are compounds that have been discovered to have anti-oxidant properties that are more powerful against a wider range of oxidants than the traditional antioxidants. They help the body detoxify, reduce inflammation, and prevent and reduce damage at the cellular level. Within this grouping, it's the flavonoid called catechin, which is found in great abundance in tea leaves, that is thought to inhibit the growth of cancerous cells. In addition to green, black, and oolong teas, flavonoids are also found in dark coloured berries, bananas, all citrus fruits, parsley, gingko biloba, and cocoa with chocolate content exceeding 70%.

Zinc: This mineral repairs damaged tissues and aids in healing wounds by generating proteins and other genetic material, boosts cell division and collagen formation, and regenerates tissue, all of which are crucial to wound repair. It boosts the system, develops and activates the T-cells that fight off infection. Zinc is found in vegetables, nuts and seeds such as asparagus, bamboo shoots, Brussels sprouts, okra, potatoes, pumpkin, Swiss chard, lima beans, peas, pine nuts, cashews, pumpkin, and sunflower seeds.

KEEPING YOUR BRAIN HEALTHY

Fernando Gómez-Pinilla, professor of neurosurgery and physiological science in UCLA, describes food as a "pharmaceutical compound that affects the brain".

Studies conducted by him show that the brain is highly susceptible to oxidation damage, so foods that are high in antioxidants protect the brain cells from damage and dysfunction.

Omega-3 fatty acids: These fatty acids support the plasticity of the synapses in the brain that affect critical functions. These include learning and memory, fighting off depression, bipolar disorders, schizophrenia, and attention-deficit disorders. The particularly important omega-3 fatty acid is docosahexaenoic acid or DHA, which reduces oxidative damage, improves synapse plasticity, and is needed in the brain's cell membranes. Omega-3s are found abundantly in walnuts, avocados, flaxseed, chia, and kiwi fruit. Though typically recommended as a desirable source of fatty acids, we take a strong stand against salmon as a source of omega-3s. The oceans are filled with toxins such as mercury, dioxin, and more recently radiation, and seafood is filled with these dangerous elements. In our annals of healing, this leads to mental and neurological disorders such as dementia, Alzheimer's, and multiple sclerosis. It is much safer and healthier to find the fatty acids in nuts and fruit.

Folic Acid: The brain needs sufficient folic acid for its functions, and folate deficiency leads to depression and cognitive impairment. Combining folic acid with other B vitamins has been effective in slowing the rate of age-related decline in cognitive function, and in preventing dementia. Folic acid is found in green leafy vegetables such as spinach, asparagus, romaine, dried or fresh beans and peas, as well as in avocados, beets, broccoli, peanuts, sunflower seeds, honeydew melons, cantaloupes, bananas, raspberries, and grapefruits.

FOODS FOR DETOXIFICATION

In our view, a good detoxification is much more than a spring-cleaning. It's like a good oil change – you take out the gunk and replace it with good, clean nutrients that power the body.

We design tailored and customized detoxification programs that both cleanse and support your system. The concept behind our programs is that it's not enough just to flush out the toxins with a juice cleanse. Instead, you need to simultaneously put back nourishment and support that will revitalize and energize the organs and the immune system.

With that being said, the key organ that is most prone to work overload is the liver. The liver supports almost every organ in the body. It is the second largest organ in the body, and any alcohol or drugs taxes it severely. When that happens, the liver performs less than optimally, leading to an accumulation of toxins that in turn cause chronic illnesses. Natural detoxification foods and herbs are best prescribed after a complete diagnosis to know what is best for your body constitution.

Natural diuretics: Foods that flush the body of toxins are essential to a good detoxification or to counteract the effects of an unhealthy lifestyle. Among natural diuretics are watercress, dandelions in the form of tea, celery, and cabbage, in which is found the antioxidant glutathione to improve the liver's detoxifying function. Be advised that natural diuretics must be used with care; the amount and type to be consumed will depend on your individual body type and constitution.

THE TRUTH ABOUT WATER

The third component to balance our Qi is water.

Water covers 71% of the Earth's surface and is vital to all forms of life. Your body ranges between 50-75% of water as body composition varies according to gender and fitness level, because adipose tissue contains less water than lean tissue. Suffering from fuzzy short-term recall, having problems with mental math or reading small print? Those are signs of dehydration. Be careful in your choice of what you drink. Tap water, sodas, and coffee are all acidic. Our rule is 8x8. We recommend drinking at least eight 8-oz. glasses of water a day to neutralize the acid in the bloodstream for better metabolism and more efficient absorption of nutrients. For those looking for alkaline water, we prefer AquaHydrate, which has a pH of 9+, but only use as directed.

"When you are sick of sickness, you are no longer sick." -Chinese proverb

149

BE AN EMPOWERED MODERN HEALER

We hope this journey into the healing properties of good nutrition will empower you to make the right choices. Whether it is to give you more energy, get you thinking clearly, accelerate recovery from illnesses, or to age with grace, the choice to eat well and live well rests in your hands. You may find the way ahead difficult and you may need a boost to get you started on the right footing. You may have inexplicable aches, pains, or chronic colds and allergies that just simply refuse to go away. Just changing your diet is not enough to get you on the healing path. Whether you seek preventative care or deep healing, we have the alternative modalities to help you with the healing transformation.

The body is a finely-tuned mechanism. It works until it is out of balance and, even then, it seeks to right itself until the imbalance has buried itself too deeply. Once it does, we are assailed with all forms of diseases and ailments, some too deep to be cured with just nutrition.

As practitioners, we tap into the secrets of our forefathers, into healing practices that have been refined and polished and provided to thousands and thousands of patients through six generations of healers. These are intricate and sophisticated methods of diagnosis, healing, and remedies that are the result of centuries of observation and practice that have withstood the tests of time and the tests of western medicine.

We are deeply immersed in a culture of healing and we drill down to the causes of disease and illness by identifying patterns of disharmony in your body. Our methods are gentle and non-invasive, and we examine not just the visible symptoms, but also take into account the subtle, intangible forces that make up all life. As healers deeply ingrained in a compassionate practice, we examine the physical, mental, emotional, and spiritual aspects because the body, mind, and spirit are inseparable. When you consult with us, you benefit not just from our knowledge and experience, but also from the cumulative wisdom and healing of our medical ancestors.

Martin and Herman are 5th and 6th generation healers steeped in Chinese healing traditions preserved through a lineage that dates back to Shaolin Buddhist principles. As father and son, they run their Toronto-based clinic on a mission to bridge the ancient and modern worlds to take healing to the next level. They seek to bring the body's energies to balance through a holistic and compassionate approach to healing. They customize nutritional plans and draw on modalities such as acupuncture and Tong Ren, a specialized energy therapy, Qi Gong breathing and exercise routines to empower the patient in the healing journey. They are currently co-authoring an upcoming book in response to overwhelming demand from their clients. It will be a thorough look at the beneficial properties, compounds, antioxidants, and micronutrients found in food, and will include ancient breathing and exercise secrets that assist in the healing process. Get more information at http://omaniclinic.com.

Coping with Cancer

YVONNE ABOU-NADER

I vividly remember the morning of April 7, 2013. I had recently moved from London and was looking to buy a house in Chelmsford to be near my sister and her family. That morning, I was drying myself after a shower when I noticed a red groove underneath my left breast. An alarm bell rang in my head as I stared at the groove. I just knew, in that moment, that I had cancer. Until then, I never noticed the groove. I was not in the habit of examining myself because I never dreamed that cancer would happen to me. I stared at the red, grooved patch and my fears ran wild as I imagined the worst.

I lived with it for ten days while waiting for an appointment with my general practitioner. I was a mess during those ten days! Confused and anxious, I was not sleeping well and could not concentrate on my work. I continuously wondered how this could have happened to me. Suddenly, the importance of conducting self-exams to feel for lumps became all too real. My last mammogram had been four years ago; I should have had one two years prior, but somehow neglected to have it done.

I strongly encourage women over the age of thirty to examine their breasts and feel for lumps. If a lump is detected, diagnosis and treatment will begin early and there will be a better chance of eradicating the cancer and preventing it from spreading to other organs, increasing the survival rate.

I kept my discovery to myself because I did not want my family to worry about me. While waiting for my appointment, I went to Chicago for my cousin's funeral. Throughout the service, I kept thinking that my turn would be next. I was terrified! Each time I undressed, the alarming red grooved patch on my breast jumped out at me. Fearing that something that looked this bad would surely be the nasty type of cancer with a low survival rate, I worried that it would be too late for successful treatment and that I would only survive a few months. Again, I kept my fears to myself and did not tell anyone.

After returning to the United Kingdom, it was time for my appointment with my general practitioner. He referred me to an oncologist who did a biopsy and scan. Two weeks later, I went back for the results of the biopsy and scan. Sitting in the waiting room, it felt like an eternity before my name was called. As time slowly passed, my mind raced with thoughts that made me even more anxious and nervous. Eventually, my name was called and I followed the nurse to the consultation room.

The oncology consultant stood up to shake my hand, indicated my chair, then waited for me to sit down. I asked him what the verdict was. He said that although he had the results of my preliminary biopsy and scan, he would need to conduct further tests. He told me that, unfortunately, he did not have good news; I had stage 3-4 breast cancer involving the lymph glands. I would need surgery before they would know the extent of my cancer.

This hit me like a ton of bricks! You can imagine how a person would react to such terrible news. The words "you have cancer" feel like a death sentence. In that moment, my world collapsed around me. Confused, shocked, angry, and scared, I repeated, "No...why me? What is happening? Why?" My first reaction was denial, even though I had heard the words I had feared all along.

HOW COULD THIS HAPPEN TO ME?

I sat there in shock and denial. What caused this? How could it happen to me? I eat the right foods and do not indulge in junk food, sugar cakes, or fizzy drinks. I do not smoke and only drink alcohol occasionally, such as one glass of wine when I go out for dinner. I exercise and work 12 hours a day, while feeling fit and well.

Upon telling me the news, the consultant realized that I was in a state of shock and asked the nurse to stay with me. She took me to a room and sat there with me, allowing me to talk and recover from the shock. I kept on repeating "Why, why?"

What had I done wrong to deserve this? What would happen to the elderly ladies who I look after and the other charitable work I do? The nurse patiently sat and listened to me vent my worries and react to the horrible news.

Once I gathered my wits, she gave me a leaflet and explained that I could get help from Macmillan nurses who specialize in cancer care in hospitals and in the community. She told me there was a telephone number if I wanted to talk to someone.

Macmillan Cancer Support is a program in the UK that offers support to people diagnosed with cancer. They understand that cancer affects every aspect of your life and work with you to help you as you deal with cancer. They can be there during treatments, they can help with job and money worries, they will listen if you just need to vent, help with benefit applications, and even offer emotional support to your whole family.

(For more info, visit www.macmillan.org.uk. It is a wonderful resource!)

On the way home from my consultation, I fixated on finding out what could be the cause of my cancer. It had not sunk in that my general practitioner had told me to stop the hormone replacement therapy (HRT). I had done this for ten years to relieve the symptoms of menopause. I eventually did stop the hormone treatments. The other contributory cause was stress, which can be an underlying cause of many diseases and illnesses. My stress level over the previous five years was enormous!

I spent the next three days on my own, not saying a word to my family or friends. Instead, I bottled up my emotions and reflected on what I could do and what action I would take. I knew I had to deal with the problem and face reality. However, I struggled to think clearly or concentrate as my mind raced with fears and worries.

On the fourth day, I called my sister and asked her to come for a visit. When she arrived, I broke the news to her and we both burst into tears. She then phoned my brother to tell him the sad news. I spoke with him and he gave me his support.

After sharing my news and allowing others to strengthen and sustain me, I was in a better place emotionally. I knew I must be positive and do the right thing to overcome the anxiety and stress so that my body could fight the cancer. I made up my mind that cancer was not going to kill me, and I would beat it no matter what it took.

WAITING FOR SURGERY

Waiting is so hard! I felt like I had to do something while waiting for my surgery, so I searched online for alternative cancer treatments in different countries. I was particularly intrigued with how cancer is treated in Japan and China. I recalled seeing a program on television about a clinic in China that treated people with cancer using natural herbs. This had also been done in Mexico with good results. I discussed these treatments with my sister and brother, along with my niece, who is a doctor. All three did not want me to go this route with my treatment.

So, I continued to wait. The ten weeks I had to wait for my surgery felt like ten years! It was an anxious and stressful time. I imagined the cancer spreading further throughout my body while I waited. I feared my prognosis would become worse with each passing day.

I carried on with my daily routine and tried to remain positive. I went to the theatre, concerts, seminars, and workshops to keep my mind occupied. I also spent time talking with friends who were always supportive and sympathetic. I continued to work three days a week so that I could be around people rather than staying home and focusing on my cancer.

Finally, it was time for my surgery. I was nervous, of course, but also strangely excited because I was going to have this invader removed from my body. When I awoke from surgery, the surgeon assured me that he removed the breast along with 14 lymph glands from under my left arm. Two of the lymph glands were large and malignant; the rest were small and nonmalignant but were sent for further tests.

After three days, I was discharged from the hospital with a drainage bag in my side, which drained excess fluid, mainly from the lymphatic system. Once I felt well enough to leave the house, I carried the drainage bag in a concealed carrier bag. I was renovating my house during this time, so I went around to the shops and bought supplies for the people working on my house. I kept myself busy so that I did not think about my situation. Then I was notified of an appointment to see the consultant to start chemotherapy.

CHEMOTHERAPY AND RADIOTHERAPY

I was told that I needed six treatments at three-week intervals, then six weeks after the chemo I would need 16 sessions of radiotherapy. I completed all the therapies, but I regret them to this day. In hindsight, I wish I had followed my gut feeling to have the surgery only. The side effects of chemotherapy and radiotherapy are not worth having them done, in my opinion. Although I do not know where I would be today if I had not had them, I would not have done these treatments had I known then what I know now.

Chemo and radiation are akin to poisoning your system. They lower your immunity, killing good cells as well as the cancer cells, and some of the side effects are irreversible. I experienced all the side effects from chemo, including losing all body hair, losing my fingernails and toenails, nausea, vomiting, loss of appetite, metallic taste (even water tasted metallic), weakness, insomnia, a burning sensation, and pain and burning on the soles of my feet. I also experienced memory loss; I knew what I wanted to say, but it would take me a couple of minutes to remember how to say it.

Additionally, I had a chest infection and neutropenic attack that required admission to the hospital for four days. My white blood cell count went down to zero! I was given antibiotics and upon discharge from the hospital, I took Vitamin B and Vitamin C supplements. I am partial to Vitamin C for building my immunity and keeping me clear of colds during the winter. I also ate nourishing fresh soup I cooked myself.

By the third week post-chemo treatment, I began to feel better. The following week I had another chemo treatment and the side effects began all over again. I ended up having only five chemotherapy sessions rather than the recommended six sessions.

FATEFUL CRUISE

Six weeks post-chemo it was time to begin radiotherapy. This took place in a different hospital which was a forty-five-minute commute from my home. My sister took me to all my radiotherapy appointments and kept me company during the treatment. The radiation burned my skin and left a lesion on my body. The side effects continue today. I suffer from a weak heart and weakened muscles.

I finished the course on the twenty-second of December and on the fourth of January I went on a cruise! I took a supply of wound dressings and anti-septic to dress the wound. I needed to get away; away from doctors and hospitals and treatments!

I flew to Miami where I got on a luxurious cruise ship called Carnival Valor. It was a magnificent ship with 11 stories. Every facility you could imagine was on board. On the ninth floor there were many restaurants with a wide variety of cuisines from different countries. There were so many choices and many different offerings, from breakfast to lunch to dinner.

The group I traveled with and I were on the second dinner seating. There were many forms of entertainment with different shows each evening; live music, comedies, interactive activities, films and even plays. I did not feel like I was on board a ship; it felt more like a city!

There were over 3,000 people on board the ship. I was traveling with a group of 450 marketers who run their own internet businesses. During one of our activities, we each had two minutes to present our line of business, the method of advertising we utilized, and our results. We had fun exchanging ideas and getting to know one another.

This group did a lot of activities together when we went ashore. We visited Mexico and stopped at the Caribbean islands, The Bahamas, and St. Antonio. I met a lot of new people and made friends that took my mind away from my cancer. I enjoyed every minute!

One day I met another woman who had the same cancer I did. She had just finished her treatment and her husband brought her on the cruise to take her mind off her ordeal and to be among people. We had an obvious, immediate bond and enjoyed sharing our stories in a positive way with each other. It was so nice to talk with someone who knew exactly what I had experienced. We were literally and figuratively in the same boat!

After the cruise, I flew to Tampa, Florida to visit with a friend before flying back to the UK. I was so inspired after the cruise that, once home, I researched alternative treatments and subscribed to cancer research institutes and health science institutes. This led me to various studies and further research on natural treatments for cancer that boast an 80-95% success rate.

MY LIFESTYLE CHANGES

I changed my diet completely and chose to follow Dr. Budwig's diet. I cut down on eating chicken, turkey, and dairy products (except for cottage cheese). I had not eaten red meat since 1986, but in the Budwig Diet you can have red meat every now and then, provided the animal is grass-fed. I continued to carry on eating freshly ground flax seeds, either with vegetable soup or mixed with quark or cottage cheese.

I also began making my own vegetable juices, using mainly organic spinach, kale, carrots, and lettuce. I ate a lot of salads and fresh fruits, including many berries: blueberries, raspberries, strawberries, and black currants. I also eat a lot of red grapes, apples, apricots, and red plums.

I bought lots of books and articles on published research about natural treatments that use diet. I have since met many people who are alive and have been cancer free for 20 years who eschewed chemo and radiation in favor of using their diet as treatment. This is, of course, a personal choice for each individual to make as each person's experiences, treatments, and outcomes will be different.

In addition to the changes I mentioned, I also eliminated sugar and artificial sweeteners; instead, I use natural stevia. I avoid many starches and carbohydrates, eating only small amounts of whole grain breads and pastas. I suggest that you avoid ready-made meals as they are usually full of preservatives. I also recommend that you avoid genetically modified foods and conventionally processed meats as the animals are often given antibiotics and fed dried foods with chemicals. I fear that these additives could cause cancer. Instead, I choose to serve fresh vegetables and organic chicken, fish, or beef.

I have since made long-term changes to my diet because I believe it may prevent my cancer from occurring again. I recently became a vegetarian and I am loving it!

In addition to diet changes, I employed other lifestyle changes as well. I try to avoid stress and worrying. That is much easier said than done! I remember how stressful it was when I discovered the mark on my breast and then later when I heard that I had cancer. Most people will remember how they felt when they were told they have cancer.

Each one of us experiences similar feelings, but each one has his or her own method for dealing with the stress and anxiety, particularly those with young children. You may experience many different emotions during your cancer diagnosis, treatment, and recovery. You may be frightened about what the future will bring to you and the effect it will have on your family. You may feel shocked and angry, as I did, but relieved to know that there is treatment available. If cancer is found and treated early, it may not be the end of your life.

There is much enjoyment to be had in life after cancer treatment. Be positive and think of a bright future ahead of you. Enjoying life to the fullest will help your progress. Have faith and believe that you will conquer cancer and live a normal life!

STRESS, DEPRESSION, AND ANXIETY

It is natural to have feelings of anxiety and/or depression when you are coping with a potentially life-threatening illness. It would be strange if you did not have these feelings! It is how you deal with it that is so important; each one of us has a way to cope with the stress and anxiety.

Anxiety can have many physical and emotional effects, from irritability, moodiness, mood swings, difficulty making decisions, memory loss, fatigue, depression, loss of appetite, and insomnia. Physical signs can include muscle tension, tightness in the chest, a racing heartbeat, and hyperventilation. When these symptoms occur simultaneously, it is called a panic attack.

I experienced most of these during my cancer treatment, but I did my best to prevent anxiety from having a drastic effect on me. I believe the cause of my cancer was the stress I had over the years before the cancer appeared. Today, I do my best to avoid any stress, which is sometimes difficult.

Stress may play a role in the onset of many diseases, particularly cancer, heart problems, and mental illnesses. Stress may reduce your life expectancy and may damage your relationship with your partner and people around you. Anxiety and stress are emotionally devastating and can lead to long-term mental illness. A study published by the American Medical Association in 2008 revealed that anxiety and stress, left untreated, can impair key areas in the brain and cause the symptoms I mentioned above. When we are stressed there will be a shortage of serotonin and Gaba compound in the body. These compounds are the body's natural anxiety and stress relievers, acting as a speed limit for the frenzied communication in the brain. Ignoring stress by brushing it under the rug and hoping it will go away on its own will not work.

When you find that anxious thoughts are taking over and preventing you from focusing on your daily life or affecting your relationship with your loved ones and the people around you, then you need to seek the help of professional people. Do not blame yourself, it is not your fault; many people feel this way. If this happens, you need to seek help from professional people. Ask your doctor to refer you to a counseling service. Most of the time it is easier to talk to a counselor rather than your family and friends. You can tell the counselor exactly how you feel without a filter and they will listen and show you empathy. They will be able to ask questions, perhaps to recall a happy memory or event, to distract you from your negative thoughts and put a smile on your face. Over time this can change the state of your mind by interrupting the negative patterns. to.

Your doctor may suggest antidepressants. I do not accept antidepressants for long-term usage. I believe that they are okay for short term usage, as you are going through a particularly stressful event, but they can be addictive and sometimes cause suicidal thoughts. There is no medical cure for anxiety or depression, only treatments. I believe you need to seek help from a qualified counselor, consider altering your diet, and make changes to your lifestyle.

TIPS FOR COPING WITH STRESS

If you continue to worry about the cancer coming back, your body may produce the same kind of stress hormone as if this were really happening. These stress hormones can cause your mind to be more anxious which results in a vicious cycle that can be difficult to break. There are several things you can do for yourself to cope with stress in addition to seeking professional help. Many of the following suggestions are simple things you can easily do for yourself, yet many of us never think of doing them. I hope you will refer to this list anytime you are feeling anxious, stress, or depressed.

- **Find a hobby:** First of all, it is important to have a healthy distraction, such as a hobby. If you do not currently have a hobby you enjoy, find one! Think of things that interest you that you can incorporate into your life, such as painting. For me, while I am painting, I shut out all negative thoughts and feelings as I focus only on what I am doing.

- **Breathing:** When you feel anxious and stressed, sit down, and take deep breaths. Inhale and exhale slowly 20 times. Imagine each intake of oxygen carrying peace and serenity to all areas of your body. With each exhale, imagine all anxiety and stress leaving your body. Accept that you cannot control everything around you. Do not aim for perfection all the time.

- **Laugh:** It has been said that laughter is the best medicine. So, watch a comedy program on television or buy tickets to see a comic perform. Welcome humor into your life; a good laugh takes your mind away from your worries.

- **Avoid negativity:** Conversely, do not invite other people's stress into your life. Do not watch the news, especially late at night. If you have a friend or family member who brings stress to you, speak with them about it. Remind them that you are in treatment or recovery and do not need any added stress. Accept that you cannot solve the world's problem. Maintain a positive attitude as you replace negative thoughts with positive thoughts.

- **Volunteer:** A terrific way to fill your mind with positive thoughts is to volunteer in your community. Helping others makes you a valuable member of the community and gives you a purpose in life. Focusing on others takes the focus off yourself and your trials. You will feel so rewarded each time you do this!

- **Find a confidante:** Talk to a friend, family member, or even someone at work. You may find a sympathetic, listening ear among your colleagues. It may be helpful for a supportive colleague to be aware of what you are going through. Talk to a member of your family or a close friend when you need to vent about your feelings or your worries. Do not get upset if friends and family tell you to just be positive and pull yourself together. Keep in mind they are simply trying to help and are probably feeling quite helpless. They will not know how you really feel; no one knows except yourself.

- **Tea time:** Drink an herbal team, such as chamomile. In addition to the calming effects of chamomile tea, the ceremony of making and drinking tea will bring about relaxation. Once it becomes a habit, you may find yourself looking forward to your cup of tea and the relaxation it brings. Drinking herbal tea before bed may promote restful sleep.

- **Visualization and meditation:** Visualization and meditation, used separately or together, will reduce stress and tension, relax the mind and body, and improve wellbeing. Lie down or sit comfortably with both feet on the floor, inhale slowly to the count of five and exhale to the count of five. Focus your attention on breathing deeply into your belly. Feel where the breath is going in your body and notice the sensation of breathing out again. For example visualize yourself lying on the beach. Now add your five senses to the picture you have created in your mind. You see the beauty of the sun, sand, and surf. Spend some time here as you picture each detail of the beach. What are you wearing? How many clouds are in the sky? Are there palm trees nearby? Once you have a vivid image of what you see, move on to what you hear. Notice the sounds of the waves crashing on the shore and the seagulls calling to each other. You are breathing the fresh air and smelling the coconut sunscreen you put on your body. You taste the saltiness of the air on your lips. Feel the gentle warmth of the sun shining on your body and the coolness of the sand underneath you. Throughout the visualization, continue your slow, steady breath. Remember to focus on breathing deeply and attend to where the breath is going in your body. If you are feeling too overwhelmed to do a full visualization on your own, listen to a relaxation podcast, calming music, or a recording of natural sounds, such as rainfall, birds singing, or ocean waves.

- **Go for a walk:** Choose a visually appealing location you enjoy and go for a brisk walk. Make it a part of your everyday routine to walk for 30 minutes or more. It will keep you fit, helping your circulation and keeping your heart healthy. You will come to look forward to your daily walk!

- **Practice yoga or Tai-Chi:** Both Tai-Chi and yoga will improve your muscle tone, flexibility, circulation, etc., while promoting relaxation and a feeling of wellbeing.

- **Eat a healthy diet:** I know I have mentioned diet previously, but I cannot emphasize enough how important it is. Unhealthy foods, smoking, and alcohol can all exacerbate stress. Many people think these things calm their stress, but it is just the opposite! Additionally, an unhealthy diet may cause other health issues. Not all alcohol is bad. A glass of red wine occasionally with the evening meal helps you relax and makes you feel sleepy. Red wine is rich in antioxidants which are beneficial to your wellbeing. Do some research to find a red wine rich with resveratrol, a beneficial antioxidant.

- **Complementary therapies:** In addition to the coping strategies for dealing with stress, there are several other complementary therapies.

These may be used alongside other treatments and include aromatherapy, reflexology, massage, music therapy, reiki, and acupuncture, to name a few.

A FAVORITE RECIPE

I have decided to share one of my personal recipes with you. This is the salad I have every day, with lunch and dinner, throughout summer and winter. I never get bored with it. I alternate some of the ingredients and buy varieties of lettuce according to the season and availability.

Yvonne's Herbal Salad

Ingredients:

- 4 leaves of lettuce (I recommend Romaine or whatever lettuce is in season where you live)
- 4 small radishes
- ¼ of a cucumber
- ½ small red onion or other onion
- 100 gm of rocket (also called arugula)
- 1 small boiled beetroot
- A few leaves of fresh mint or dried mint
- ½ freshly squeezed lemon
- 1 clove of garlic minced or chopped

- 3 tablespoon of extra virgin olive oil or organic flaxseed oil

- A pinch of salt

Method:

1. Wash all lettuces and vegetables under cool running water.

2. Chop the lettuce, radish, cucumber, rocket, beetroot, and onion and place in a bowl.

3. Mix the mint, lemon, garlic, oil, and salt together. Pour over the vegetables and enjoy.

Additions and Alterations:

Occasionally, maybe once a month, I add 40 gm of feta cheese to the salad. Other times I may add black olives. I sometimes change up the vegetables I use, depending on what is in season. I may use baby-leaf spinach mixed with rocket and omit the cucumber. I sometimes add a small tomato and grated carrot. I may use fresh thyme or dill, when in season.

I also like to add freshly boiled red kidney beans on occasion. I soak dried beans overnight and boil in the morning to use in my salad later in the day. (I never buy tin food, as it is full of sugar, salt, and preservatives.)

Other times I use boiled chickpeas in the salad. Or, I make them as a dip to enjoy on the side. I mash the chickpeas with added lemon juice, olive or flaxseed oil, garlic, onion, and mint. I enjoy this as a side with my salad.

I concluded that what you eat matters to your health to maintain your immune system and lead a healthy life. I hope you enjoy this recipe and that it inspires you to create other healthy options. If you would like to have more recipes and learn what to eat and do to remain healthy, build your immune system, and boost your energy, send me an email at naderyvonne@yahoo.com

Purpose and Living Your Passion Cure

RON BELL

This chapter is about Ron Bell's defining your *Purpose and living your Passion Cure*. It offers 10 powerful ways to discover true inner peace and happiness. However, in order to understand each step in this process, we need to begin with two basic definitions.

First we'll look at the word purpose. Purpose is the reason for which something is done or created or for which something exists. Some useful synonyms are motive, motivation, cause, occasion, reason, basis, justification. When used as a verb, purpose is one's intention or objective. It has such synonyms as: intend, mean, aim, plan, design, decide, resolve, determine, propose, aspire. For example, I know someone who gets up every morning and purposefully begins to work on his goals at 6 am. He does not stop until 4 pm. He has a plan, the resolve to fulfill it and the motivation to meet all challenges. In other words, while his day is filled with purpose he also has a purpose.

Next we'll define the word passion. Passion is strong and barely a controllable emotion. The man in the previous example works, plays and rests on purpose. He is driven. The emotions he feels are strong, sometimes barely controllable; he needs to move through his days with a sense of purpose, resolve and determination. He is filled with passion.

The first question that begs to be asked, of course, is how do you get to such a place? How do you get on purpose and become motivated to stay there? One step is to begin with an inventory of your strengths. The way to do this is to ask yourself a series of questions. Ask yourself a question and the mind will always answer. Always. For example: Are you loyal? Do you pursue your assignments with pertinacity? Why do you act the way you do when faced with difficulty? Are you courageous? Honest? What are your greatest assets? Write your answers down on a piece of blank paper. Do you act on purpose throughout the day? How about passion—do you act with and feel great emotion that drives you forward toward your purpose, a passion that takes your strengths and carries them toward perfection? Create a list of the resources you, as an individual, possess and that you can get behind both mentally and emotionally.

There's wisdom in knowing your strengths: Men or women who know their strengths are never without resources. They can turn to this tool box whenever some difficulty or trouble passes through their lives. Your strengths can be the difference between staying on task (or purpose) and falling back into the rut that most people live in. This is why it's so important to combine purpose and passion. Acting on purpose from minute to minute depends completely on your motivation, and your motivation is very much about passion. The greater your emotional investment in your action, the greater will be that which drives you. Think of passion as the gas that runs the car of purpose. You can't go anywhere on an empty tank. Similarly, you can't run on gas tainted by water. You will eventually falter and stall, placing you right back where you used to be. Yes, purpose and passion go hand in hand.

Now for the *10 powerful ways to discover true inner peace and happiness:*

STEP 1: EMBRACE CHANGE

Did you know that the average person hates change? In fact, they spend their lives trying to build cocoons to keep change at bay. Little do they know that, like the butterfly, we are a chrysalis that is turned into a human version of the butterfly by the pressure of change. If, in your life, you are receiving the same results, you must change what you are doing. Then and only then will you receive a different result. Knowing this, shouldn't we learn to embrace change? Get serious about it! Determine what your natural gifts and talents are. This list will be different than the one you made regarding your strengths. This list is about the thing(s) you know, without a doubt, that you are better at than anyone else. In fact it's probably the one single and natural thing you dream about spending your life doing. (Your true Passion).

How do you begin working on using the strengths and talents you've found to create positive changes in your life? The answer is, become conscious of the choices you make on a moment-to-moment basis. Create awareness of what it is you are thinking, saying and doing throughout your day. Then begin to make these choices on purpose and with passion.

Part of making positive change in your life is identifying your dreams. Your dreams will probably rotate around those gifts or talents you discovered a few steps back. For example, somewhere within that dream vacation is also a dream of how you came to be there. What is your dream job? Why? How can you achieve it? I'll tell you how ....

Once you've clearly identified your dreams, you need to understand that turning them into reality is all about goal setting. It requires that you reverse engineer those big dreams, breaking them down until you arrive at some task you can do today and in the days to come.

Stay disciplined and focused. Once you begin setting daily goals it's very important that you stay disciplined. No weekdays off or early check-outs for you. True goal-setting requires that you spend your day focused on each goal you apply yourself to—one at a time, hour by hour and day by day—until you reach that far away dream which can create and inner peace and true happiness.

STEP 2: FIND PURPOSE AND PASSION

Self-empowerment is the actuation of the self through minute-to-minute choices. These are choices made on purpose, with real focus and passion. It's the result of knowing your strength and your dreams and having a plan, through goal-setting, to use those strengths to get there.

However, all these changes can increase your stress levels. Happily, the way to decrease stress is to take the task at the top of your prioritized list of goals and put all your focus on it, never thinking of any of the other tasks on your list until you have finished the one you are currently working on—even if you don't finish your list of daily goals. In such a case they just get added to the next day's list. Why does this work? It works because it eliminates worry (most likely one of your biggest stressors). It will also let you get more done than any other system you might happen to try.

I'll tell you a secret. The system of goal-setting I've been talking about will create a new zest for life in you, and it will leave you happier. Why? You'll have virtually eliminated worry in your life. Secondly, our minds are goal-oriented machines. By creating a focused plan, you'll be tapping into that problem-solving aspect of your mind, and it will leave you satisfied at the end of each day. A person who is satisfied with where they are in life and with whatever they have will generally be happier.

Lifestyle change, which is huge and what most individuals desire, will come as you change the decisions you make throughout the day. Make the conscious choice to make positive decisions leading to your goals. Make an extra sale a week, 50 more telephone calls per week, or take on more responsibility at work—all these changes tend to lead to lifestyle changes. So can your daily decisions: the choice to not go for a coffee break at the local café puts more money in your pocket every day; the simple choice to smile in the moment can bring all sorts of changes to your life as you meet new people and enamour the ones you know. The list is endless. Change your moment-to-moment choices and watch your life alter before your eyes.

As you become a more confident decision-maker and an even more stellar goal-setter, you'll undoubtedly notice that your personal confidence will grow exponentially. There's something about making the right choices and doing the right things (for you) that boosts people's confidence immensely.

And … you may never work again. This point may seem silly to you, but it holds a kernel of truth. When you begin to act on purpose, pursuing goals designed to bring you your greatest dreams, you'll find that you're no longer working but rather you're having fun and experiencing happiness. You'll be filled with a passion for action. No longer will problems plague you, because you'll know that each problem solved takes you a step closer to the fulfilment of your daily goals and your ultimate dreams.

STEP 3: SEVERAL INTERTWINED METHODS FOR OBTAINING INNER PEACE

One way to obtain inner peace is to go in deep with meditation. There are many different forms of meditation, and it's beyond the scope of this piece to point you in a specific direction. Suffice it to say that meditation serves two purposes: 1) to clear the mind and 2) to create an intense feeling of focus and well-being. By going deep into a meditative state you can face whatever it is that lies before you with a renewed sense of passion and clarity of thought. Sounds good doesn't it?

Joining up and networking with individuals who are on a "passion" quest for the gift or talent that will light a fire beneath them like never before is heady stuff and very important. You must surround yourself with "like" minded individuals. These are people who are excited by the prospect of finally discovering and doing what they were born to do. They're a special club of people who are passionately working on achieving their dreams. And that excitement will rub off on you. I am personally involved with a Success Training Company called PEAK POTENTIALS. If you would personally like to take your life to the next level, I recommend you attend their self-development seminar. It's a true life-changing event. You may register at: http://lifepurposeandpassionbook.com/ -- a great group of people to rub shoulders with! You've got to know this will lead to greater inner peace.

Fasting is a biblical way to truly humble yourself in the sight of God (Psalm 35:13; Ezra 8:21). King David said, "I humble myself through fasting."

Fasting can transform your prayer life into a richer and more personal experience. Fasting can also result in a dynamic personal revival in your own life and can make you a channel of revival to others. It most definitely leads to inner peace.

And finally, self-reflection, like fasting, can clear your mind. Serious thought about one's character, actions, and motives can bring a sense of cohesiveness that can't help but create a greater sense of peace.

STEP 4: DISCOVER YOUR LIFE PURPOSE

Many people never discover their "life purpose." They get caught up in earning a living, raising a family and a thousand other different things. They might play wistfully with a hobby they love or they might daydream about doing something they secretly think would bring them the true contentment they desire. But they never quite reach the point where they make the jump to living their dreams.

The truth of the matter is that *Success is … taking action.* One must become actively aware of what it is that they were put on this earth to do. You know what this is. It's that secret dream you hardly dare to dream of. Or it's something people have always said you were born to do. Whatever your gift or talent is, deep down you know it. You just need to bring it to the forefront of your mind, you need to seek true awareness. Next comes action. The average person never takes enough small steps to create the momentum needed to move forward into the life of their dreams. Success is … taking action. Break your dreams down into ever smaller tasks until you reach the point where you have a list of things you can do now—today. Act on them.

[1]http://www.cru.org/train-and-grow/devotional-life/personal-guide-to-fasting.2.html

Take the thousand baby steps that will add up to massive action. Begin right now. The number of people who begin the journey to their dreams but never get there are countless. It's not their fault. They never knew that they had to carefully analyze their actions. A ship gets to its destination by making the minute-to-minute analysis of its position and then making course adjustments necessary to stay moving in the direction of the targeted port of call. Do not try to "eat" the whole elephant. Focus and take small steps to reach the bigger goal. Take realistic steps to reach your goals and obtain your dreams because, when you make unrealistic goals, you set yourself up for frustration and ultimately failure. People must chase their dreams in the same way. We must constantly adjust what we do to make sure we stay on the right path.

You might think this path will be too stressful. And stress can kill. Everyone knows that. Well, if you don't want stress then you must first accept that happiness, joy, contentment and beauty are the natural order of things. Did you know that 47% of all cancer cases is due to "pent up anger and resentment? Strive for continued happiness. It may be a stretch at first, because I can almost guarantee you don't have these things in your daily life. It's not your fault. Chances are no one ever taught you how to consciously focus on bringing them into your daily life. That's right: the key to removing stress from your life is to purposely bring happiness, joy, contentment and beauty into your life by making the right choices on a minute-to-minute basis. It's that simple and that difficult. But you can do it. I know you can.

You really must choose the environments mentioned above. Toxic environments kill everything in their path. You must choose to live differently, every minute of your life. And you can't expect to be valued if you don't, first, value yourself. Change your thinking and your actions will change, and people will sense it. They will look at you differently. Because we are, most definitely what we think. The Process of Manifestation is: Thoughts lead to Feelings.

Feelings lead to Actions. Actions lead to Results. Let's get Positive RESULTS in our lives!! Your inner thoughts will determine your outer world!

STEP 5: LEARN TO THINK POSITIVELY

Many people think that positive thinking implies seeing the world through rose-colored lenses, and ignoring or glossing over the negative aspects of life. You know—the glass is half full instead of half empty. However, positive thinking actually means approaching life's challenges with a positive outlook. It does not necessarily mean avoiding or ignoring the bad things; instead, it involves making the most of potentially bad situations, trying to see the best in other people, and viewing yourself and your abilities in a positive light. Such habits reduce stress and increase your level of contentment and happiness.

Why is positive thinking contagious? This is what I call a "no brainer." Who would you rather hang out with: the guy who is always the life of the party or the grumpy guy in the next cubicle at work? The choice is obvious, right? But why is it obvious? It's obvious because the guy who's the life of the party makes you feel good—about the party and about yourself. And therein lies the key. If you alter how you view yourself and your abilities, other people will alter their behaviours regarding you. Call it the psychology of the masses or some other technical term: it doesn't change the fact that, in general, people respond to us based on how we see ourselves.

How can you turn negative thinking into positive thinking? Positive thinking must be made a habit for it to work. That means you must be willing to consciously choose your thoughts or your response to what is going on in your life from a minute-to-minute standpoint, until the process becomes second nature. This takes commitment and hard work, something most people aren't going to do for a process they don't even understand. But you now understand, don't you?

An example of positive thinking: "The history of the baby frog.......

Once upon a time there was a bunch of baby frogs....

... participating in a competition. The target was to get to the top of a high tower. A crowd of people had gathered to observe the race and encourage the participants.....

The start shot rang out.......

Quite honestly:

None of the onlookers believed that the baby frogs could actually accomplish getting to the top of the tower.

They said things like:"Åh, it's too difficult!!!

They'll never reach the top."

or: "Not a chance... the tower is too high!"

One by one some of the baby frogs fell off...

...Except those who quickly climbed higher and higher..

The crowd kept on yelling:

"It's too difficult. Nobody is going to make it!"More baby frogs became tired and gave up...

...But one kept going higher and higher.....

He was not giving up!

At the end everybody had given up, except the one determined to reach the top! All the other participants naturally wanted to know how he had managed to do what none of the others had been able to do!

One competitor asked the winner, what was his secret?

The truth was.......

The winner was deaf!!!!

The lesson to be learned:

Don't ever listen to people who are negative and pessimistic...

...they will deprive you of your loveliest dreams and wishes you carry in your heart! Always be aware of the power of words, as everything you hear and read will interfere with your actions!

Therefore:

Always stay...

POSITIVE!

And most of all:

Turn a deaf ear when people tell you that you cannot achieve your dreams!

Always believe:

You can make it! Stay Positive!!!

STEP 6: ELIMINATE NEGATIVITY

Until you've become strong enough to be able to ward off the negativity in situations it would be a great idea to avoid watching the news. It might even be good to avoid television altogether. Why? Because there's so much that is negative or that will counter your attempts to live a contented and happy lifestyle that it could severely hamper your efforts.

Just to make a point. I turned on the television last night when I got home, and set about having a relaxing evening. There were at least six channels that were talking about current terrorism threats and many other channels were carrying shows full of violence and bloodshed. Tell me how that works to help you change your mindset in a positive way? I'm not saying not to watch television, but be very careful what you put into your psyche.

What was said previously goes double for negative environments. If a situation truly is negative, how do you expect to truthfully change your thoughts about it? You can do it, but you'll most likely be kidding yourself. The way to stay positive, contented and happy is to make certain your day is filled with light and beauty, not darkness and ugliness. Make sense?

Adopt healthy eating habits. Is thinking about having a hamburger and French fries for lunch really bad thinking? It is if you're overweight and your goal is to lose that weight. To adopt healthy eating habits (and this goes for anyone, not just the overweight), one must make those moment-to-moment positive choices we've been talking about. The choice to choose a salad over a hamburger and fries is simple—if you are acting on "purpose."

Focus on the "whats" not the "what ifs." What can I do about my current situation to make it a positive and joyful experience? What if this wasn't happening to me? What if I just skipped out? What if I made the effort to enjoy myself? Which of these questions will make certain my thoughts and actions are going to ensure the best possible experience? If you chose question the first one, then you're beginning to get the hang of "positive thinking." Do not look at opportunities and situations in life and say, "I'll believe it when I see it". You will miss opportunities over and over again. It's the exact opposite, YOU WILL SEE IT WHEN YOU BELIEVE IT" Have Faith! Just because you do not see the seeds growing, doesn't mean, they are not growing. Please refer to the story of the Chinese Bamboo Tree—the story of patience.

What do you love? What do you love to do? I'm not just talking about work here. What leisure activities do you love? What can you do to make sure you build as many of these activities into your days as possible? Remember the goal-setting process? By placing leisure activities on your priority list, you'll be sure to do them when their turn arrives. If I've booked a tee time at my favourite golf course for 2 pm, then I know my workday is going to end at two, and I can prioritize my daily to-do list accordingly, knowing that no matter what happens I will quit working at that time.

Will such practices work every time? Of course not. Life is full of problems and obstacles. But I can guarantee that such habits will bring more pleasure and inner peace into your life than any other method I know of.

STEP 7: DEVELOP YOUR "SELF"

The threat to your continued self-development is inaction. Regardless of the reason or excuse, you can't change anything about your life unless you take purposeful, massive action. Those countless moment-to-moment choices that lead to action of unimaginable proportions must be made on purpose and with specific results in mind. Failure to do this consistently is the one major threat to the achievement of anything you want—include self-development. Best Selling Author T. Harv Eker was quoted saying, "Rich Minded People continue to learn and Grow and Poor "minded" and Middle Class people think that they already know." It's key to invest in your continuous self-development.

Find a life coach. Why do you need a life coach? A person who has already done the things you want to do can guide you past the many pitfalls that lie before you. She can also ensure that you make the right moment-to-moment decisions. She's been there, remember? A successful life coach can shorten your journey by years. Isn't that worth the investment of money and effort? I think it is.

Associate with like minds. People have the ability to affect others through changes in their mindset and their actions. Imagine what could happen if like-minded people came together. The effect could be explosive. I know for a fact that two like-minded people can increase their success exponentially. It's like they form a third mind, a "mastermind," that lifts them up and carries them forward. The effect increases as you add more people to your group. You can even have more than one mastermind group. Some will focus on personal development, some on work and some on investing. You can have a mastermind group for just about any aspect of your life. Anytime two or more like-minded people get together great things can happen.

Read self-help books. Again, you can benefit from those who have gone before you. There are thousands of self-help books out there. And they cover just about any subject you can imagine. Invest in them. There isn't any rule that says your mentor must be a live person. Books can and do teach people how to attain their goals in life.

Enrol in self-development programs. Dale Carnegie, perhaps the greatest motivator ever, taught many, many thousands of people how to achieve their dreams. His books touched many others. His speaking courses were genius in motion. Enrolling in similar courses can give each of us the spark to move forward, to take action with a purpose. You don't have to do this thing alone. Find a program to help you along.

Everything that has been laid down in this outline could be considered the process by which you can change your character and/or your abilities for the better. Don't you think that such positive changes would make you happier and more at peace with yourself? All that remains is for you to take action.

STEP 8: LEARN THE LAW OF ATTRACTION

The law of attraction is the name given to the term that "like attracts like" and that by focusing on positive or negative thoughts, one can bring about positive or negative results. This belief is based upon the idea that people and their thoughts are both made from "pure energy" and the belief that like energy attracts like energy. One example used by a proponent of the law of attraction is that if a person opened an envelope expecting to see a bill, then the law of attraction would "confirm" those thoughts and contain a bill when opened. A person who decided to instead expect a cheque might, under the same law, find a cheque instead of a bill. Although there are some cases where positive or negative attitudes can produce corresponding results, there is no scientific basis to the law of attraction.

How to use the Law of Attraction and how it may assist you: "The one who speaks most about illness has illness. The one who speaks about prosperity has prosperity," Esther and Jerry Hicks write. "You attract all of it." By focusing on something, you make it happen. And oh how true this is. In life focus can be everything. Think about something long enough and hard enough and you're sure to become attuned to actions that can make it happen. The intense focus will also increase the chances that you will act on your thoughts when the opportunity presents itself.

It's very easy for people who know this secret to believe that like attracts like, but I caution against that belief. What is actually happening is you are becoming more alert to and more ready to take the actions that will lead to whatever it is you want. Make enough such choices and you are almost certain to arrive at your destination. And it can really feel like magic!

Successful people know many of the things I've been writing about. They know that if they put themselves out there they will eventually bump into something like they are looking for, whether that's a person, a place, or a thing. It's all about focus and the choices that result.

The old adages are that we reap what we sow, that what goes around comes around and that what we give so shall we receive. The whole point is that our focus/choice combination works every way. Put your focus on giving something different to your community or to your family and you will tend to make choices that will reflect that change in thinking. The changes will be noticed by others, who you can be certain will eventually return the favour however they can. It's a great way to live and you can reap rewards beyond your imagination.

STEP 9: TAKE YOUR QUALITY OF LIFE TO THE NEXT LEVEL

There is nothing so strong and so life-affirming as love. Felice Leonardo "Leo" Buscaglia PhD (March 31, 1924 – June 12, 1998), also known as "Dr. Love," was an American author and motivational speaker, and a professor in the Department of Special Education at the University of Southern California. He believed that, the more you love, the greater becomes your capacity for love, a rather contrary vision of what love is like. This was a view of love as having the infinite power to change us and those around us. In fact he said as much in the following quote: *Too often we underestimate the power of a touch, a smile, a kind word, a listening ear, an honest compliment, or the smallest act of caring, all of which have the potential to turn life around.* – Leo Buscaglia

I could go a step further and say that the greatest phenomenon in the universe is the concept of love. Many see God as love. A fact I know is that the more you give love, the more you tend to receive, whether you're thinking of God or yourself or another. Yes, self-love is important. We can only love our God or our spouse or anyone else as much as we love ourselves. How can it be any different? We can only give what we have and what we know.

This also goes for the intensity of our love. It is our deep belief and our intensity that gives us the power to affect others. For this reason it is a worthwhile exercise to practice intensity of love.

I also admonish you to give as you hope to receive. We have all heard this platitude. It has lost what power it might ever have had. But this does not diminish the truth. If you are willing to sacrifice to give to another or to your community, then you fundamentally change yourself. You become more willing to help, to put yourself out there. People will remember this. So, when the time comes when you are in need, as we all are at some point in life, you'll find that all your sacrifices will be remembered and returned tenfold. It may not be in the way you expect, but it will happen. There's too much anecdotal evidence to believe otherwise.

And as I close, love once again comes into play. Open your heart to the universe and it will fill you up. Give all this back and you will feel as you have never felt before. Some call it a religious conversion, others refer to it as enlightenment; still others speak of a sense of peace and happiness. The bottom line is that you can't love too much. It's impossible. Love can't be used up, so don't be afraid to reach out (take action) for what is waiting for you. You won't regret it.

STEP 10: MORE WAYS TO FIND TRUE INNER PEACE

Apologize and Forgive – When a person apologizes for a wrong he's done or forgives a wrong done unto her an amazing thing happens. All the negative thoughts and emotions you were harbouring simply melt away. You may want to know why this is the case. The answer is incredibly simple: you change your focus. Your moment-to-moment thoughts and actions turn away from what was bothering you and suddenly things are new again.

Relax – Inner peace is a state created by you. Taking time out of your busy day to just relax and allow your mind to drift away to your favourite destinations is a good place to start.

Be Grateful – Happiness and contentment come from being grateful for what you already have. Take your focus and place it on thoughts and actions that indicate to you that you are, indeed, grateful.

Go outdoors – Nature is the great healing balm. A walk in the forest, a stroll through your garden, a ride on your bike or any other outside activity that gets your body moving and breathing in fresh air can't help but improve your disposition.

Go Inside Yourself – The best way I know to go inside myself is meditation, which is the practicing of certain techniques that allow you to clear your mind, heighten your focus and then point your mind in the direction you wish to go.

Know When to Stand Firm – Inner peace is sometimes reached by facing down a problem, whether that be an intense short-term task or a longer-term worry. Face down your problems, find the best way to deal with them, do those things and then forget about them. Inner peace will be yours.

Learn the Power of Surrender – When people talk about surrendering they're usually talking about God. There's something amazingly powerful about giving up yourself and your problems to the holy spirit. I think the largest part of this is that you are giving up all your worries. Joe Tye (CEO and Head Coach of Values Coach Inc., which provides consulting, training and coaching on values-based life and leadership skills.) once said "Worry is ingratitude to God in advance." Think about that for a moment!

Be the Love You Want to Feel – If you want to feel loved, then you must not only love yourself but demonstrate your love for others. It's a risky thing to do—putting yourself out there like that—but you already know that we reap what we sow.

Be of Service – Strange things (good things) happen when you give of yourself to your community, the first of these being a sense of belonging, which goes a long way to creating inner peace.

Be Here Now – And, finally, making the choice to be in the moment, to enjoy each and every one we have during our time on earth, creates such a sense of joy that one soon relaxes and finds a sense of inner peace. Try it, you'll see.

[2]http://www.thebridgemaker.com/10-paths-to-true-happiness/

www.ingramcontent.com/pod-product-compliance
Lightning Source LLC
Chambersburg PA
CBHW072227270326
41930CB00010B/2027